The New Genetics and the Public's Health

The rapid advancement of genetic science, fuelled by the Human Genome Project and other related initiatives, promises a new kind of public health practice based on the pre-detection of disease according to calculations of genetic risk. This book by two well-known sociologists:

- explores the implications of the new genetics for public health as a body of knowledge and a domain of practice;
- assesses the impact of new genetic information and technologies on conceptions of health, illness, embodiment, self and citizenship;
- critically examines the complex discourses surrounding human genetics and public health;
- discusses the role of the media in framing debate about genetics, health and medicine.

The New Genetics and the Public's Health addresses the emerging social and political consequences of the new genetics and provides a stimulating critique of current research and practice in public health.

Alan Petersen is Professor in Sociology of Health and Illness at the University of Plymouth. **Robin Bunton** is Reader in Social Policy, University of Teesside.

The New Genetics and the Public's Health

Alan Petersen
and Robin Bunton

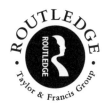

London and New York

First published 2002
by Routledge
11 New Fetter Lane, London EC4P 4EE

Simultaneously published in the USA and Canada
by Routledge
29 West 35th Street, New York, NY 10001

Routledge is an imprint of the Taylor & Francis Group

© 2002 Alan Petersen and Robin Bunton

Typeset in Times New Roman by Taylor & Francis Books Ltd
Printed and bound in Great Britain by TJ International Ltd,
Padstow, Cornwall

British Library Cataloguing in Publication Data
A catalogue record for this book is available from the British
Library

Library of Congress Cataloging in Publication Data
Petersen, Alan R., Ph. D.
The new genetics and the public's health / Alan Petersen and
Robin Bunton.
Includes bibliographical references and index.
1. Medical genetics–Social aspects. 2. Human genetics–Social
aspects. I. Bunton, Robin, 1954– II. Title.

RB 155 .P48 2001
616'.042–dc21
 2001048171

ISBN 0–415–22141–2 (hbk)
ISBN 0–415–22142–0 (pbk)

Contents

Acknowledgements

Alan Petersen would like to thank the following people who have assisted by way of generously offering items of information: Dr Patricia Spallone, Dr Sarah Cunningham-Burley, Professor Peter Glasner, Dr Tom Shakespeare, Dr Christopher Newell, Dr Paul Martin, Dr Lene Koch, Dr Nina Hallowell, Professor Elizabeth Ettorre, Professor Nicholas Rose, Professor Peter Conrad, and Professor Waqar Ahmad. He wishes to thank delegates at the Ethos of Welfare Conference in Finland in August 2000, and at the BSA Medical Sociology Conference in York, UK, in September 2000, who provided feedback on some work in progress which provided the basis for some of his chapters. He is also grateful to participants at the Workshop on the Ethical, Social and Legal Implications of the Human Genome Project, held in Adelaide, South Australia, in December 2000, who offered numerous useful insights, and to Professor Riaz Hassan, who invited him to participate. Murdoch University was generous in offering a six-month period of study leave in 2000, which allowed him to write part of the book. Finally, he wishes to thank his partner, Ros Porter, who is a constant source of companionship and support.

Some of the material which appears in Chapter 4 is reprinted from *Social Science and Medicine*, 52, 8 (2001), Alan Petersen, 'Biofantasies: genetics and medicine in the print news media', pages 1255–68, with permission from Elsevier Science. Material appearing in Chapter 5 is a development of ideas originally published in Alan Petersen, 'Counselling the genetically "at risk": the poetics and politics of "non-directiveness"', *Health, Risk and Society* (http://www.tandf.co.uk), 1, 3 (1999): 253–65.

Robin Bunton extends thanks to a number of people who have supported and discussed this project, including Pamela Abbott and members of the Sociology section in the School of Social Sciences, University of Teesside, who made it possible for him to take study leave to support the research for this project. Thanks, too, to Barbara Cox, who provided vital administrative support throughout (as well as a sense of humour) and to Paul Crawshaw for his interest and sharing of ideas and leads. Thanks to Gary Wickham and colleagues in the School of Social Inquiry, Murdoch University, Western Australia, for their support and debate at the time of researching this book. Thanks also to Ann Robertson and her colleagues at the University of Toronto, who provided interesting debate in the latter stages of this project, and similarly to Ron Labonte and his colleagues at the Universities of Regina and Saskatoon. Thanks to Richard Hardesty and Maggie Tebb for excellent food and feisty arguments over the period of writing. Finally, thanks to Lesley Jones for her continued intellectual support and sense of proportion.

Both Alan Petersen and Robin Bunton wish to thank Heather Gibson, who as previous Senior Editor at Routledge encouraged us to collaborate in the writing of this book. Edwina Welham, current Senior Editor, was generous in offering assistance during the final stages and in granting an extension for the completion of the manuscript.

Alan Petersen wishes to dedicate his contributions to this book to his father, Neil Petersen, who died as this book was being completed. Without his love and support, and that of his mother, Gwen Petersen, he would never have had the opportunity to write books.

Chapter 1

Introduction

The new genetics, health, and 'the public'

Alan Petersen

This book explores the applications of new genetic knowledge for the health of 'the public', and the way these are changing how we think about our bodies, ourselves, and society. It examines how genetics is shaping our conceptions of the natural and the normal, and what are seen as the possibilities for treatment, prevention, and cure. The impact of new genetic knowledge, we contend, extends from the local level to the global level. It not only affects how we, individually, view our bodies, our selves, and our families, but also shapes our social relations across national borders. New genetic knowledge is emerging in the context of, and is contributing to, a redefinition of the relationship between citizens and the state, accompanying the increasing liberalization of markets and transnational flows of information and economic exchanges. The findings of genetic research are being rapidly applied in practices of population screening, diagnostic testing, and counselling, and promise to revolutionize the treatment of disease through the development of new therapies and drugs, profoundly affecting personal and social life. Indeed, developments in this area bring into question the very notions of the person and society. In the book we identify the diverse imperatives associated with these new genetic technologies, and indicate how they are affecting the lives of everyone. We begin, in this chapter, by outlining the book's perspective and guiding assumptions, and introducing the chapters that follow.

Our perspective can be described, broadly, as a sociocultural perspective, in that we examine the social and cultural contexts within which the field of 'public health genetics' is emerging, and takes meaning. This sets it apart from the perspectives of medical genetics, preventive medicine, and much of bioethics, which dominate the literature on genetics and human health. In recent years, there has been an outpouring of new texts focusing on new genetic findings and their medical applications, and exploring the attendant ethical and legal implications. Much of this work has arisen against a background of recent 'gene-mapping' initiatives such as the Human Genome Project (HGP), which are seen to give rise not only to medical possibilities of previously unimaginable dimensions, but also to major ethical and legal dilemmas. Although such work is often insightful and thought-provoking, it tends to leave unexamined the broader social and cultural contexts within which new genetic ideas arise, assume meaning, and are applied. Science is seen as essentially separate from, or outside, society rather than as a social product. Genetic knowledge is viewed as an outcome of scientists' objective search for the 'facts', which are then taken up by, and impact on, 'society' in various ways. There is little recognition of how culture affects the content and practice of science: what is defined as a problem, how research is undertaken, what counts as a fact, and how findings are communicated and applied. Questions concerning the power relations of science, and the relationship between power and knowledge, are left largely unexamined. That such work tends to be unreflective about, and uncritical of, science and its power relations is hardly surprising since it is contributed largely by scientists themselves, who have a vested interest in sustaining a particular definition of genetics and its benefits. However, non-scientists, including journalists who report on new genetic discoveries, also frequently share the assumption that science and society are essentially separate.

We are not the first to adopt a sociocultural perspective on new genetic technologies, particularly as they are applied in the area of health. During the 1990s, a growing number of scholars in the social sciences and humanities turned their attention to questions such as the social construction and meanings of genetic knowledge, and lay people's uptake of, and responses to, information provided by experts such as genetic counsellors. (Recent social science books include Conrad and Gabe, 1999a; Kaplan, 2000; Katz Rothman, 1998; Keller, 2000; O'Sullivan et al., 1999; Rapp, 1999). Some of this work does critically examine science and its social contexts and impacts. For example, sociological work explores reproductive genetics as an aspect of surveillance medicine and body management (Ettorre, 1996, 2000), the new human genetics as a feature of 'reflexive modernity' (Kerr and Cunningham-Burley, 2000), and lay perspectives on genetics, inheritance, and risk (Kerr et al., 1998a,

1998b). However, previous work has been limited largely to examining the influence of genetic ideas on specific areas of health care or public health, such as new technologies of genetic screening or prenatal genetic diagnosis, rather than exploring the broad impacts of genetic ideas and technologies on conceptions of self and society. It has also tended to view genetic knowledge and its applications in isolation from changing politico-economic and global contexts. There has been little appreciation of how these contexts shape our thinking and action in relation to genetics and its applications in public health. In this book, we highlight the significance of these contexts, showing how new genetic knowledge is reshaping conceptions of health, disease, and normality. On the one hand, we are interested in the ways in which genetics is transforming public health as a body of knowledge and a domain of practice, and in exploring what this means for how we think about the individual and society. On the other, we are concerned with how appeals to the 'health' of 'the public' are shaping responses to those who have been diagnosed with a genetic condition or are deemed to be genetically 'at risk', and are affecting people's views of their bodies, selves, and relationships. We examine constructions of 'the public', and of medicine, science, and technology, and how these advantage a particular viewpoint on genetics and its applications.

Beginning in this chapter, and in the chapter that follows, we examine the nature of the new expertise, institutions and practices developed as a consequence of the increasing focus on genetic health and disease, and assess the implications for the ordering and regulation of personal and social life. We show how genetics is defining new domains for analysis and intervention, resulting in a shift in the distribution of material and financial resources. We ask: what does genetics imply in terms of how we consider the concept of 'public health', which traditionally has been defined in terms of population, and changing those external environmental conditions which predispose people to disease? To what extent, and in what ways, does the focus on molecular biology challenge established understandings of 'the environment' and of population health? What are the political and practical implications of the effort to incorporate new genetic ideas into the strategies and practices of public health? And, are the promises of the new genetic-based public health (e.g. increased choice, improved health) likely to be fulfilled? An assessment of how genetics is shaping the domain of public health should involve consideration of the impact of genetic knowledge and practice on people's everyday lives and relationships. We ask: what do such developments mean for people's views of their own bodies, concept of self, experience of illness, and sense of wellbeing, and for how they conduct themselves, interact with others, and plan their lives? Who has access to the new genetic technologies, and is there any potential for inequalities to arise as a result of the widespread uptake of genetic knowledge in public health? What scope is there for people to contest the imperatives surrounding genetic-based public health?

This book arises out of our shared interest in exploring the implications of genetics for the understanding and analysis of contemporary public health. It builds on previous work, which entails a critical analysis of the knowledge and practices of health promotion and public health, and associated forms of social regulation (Bunton *et al.*, 1995; Petersen and Bunton, 1997; Petersen and Lupton, 1996). Influenced by recent trends in social thought, particularly the insights offered by 'governmentality' scholars, we have explored the inextricable links between dominant conceptions of the person and their dispositions and actions and a prevailing form of rule in contemporary societies, variously known as 'neo-liberalism' or 'advanced liberalism'. Although the defining features of this rule are the subject of ongoing debate, there is broad agreement among writers that advanced liberalism operates not so much through coercive means as through creating conditions that allow people to govern themselves. In advanced liberal societies, authorities recognize that it is usually much easier to achieve governmental goals if citizens believe that they are in charge of their own destinies, that their actions are unconstrained, and that they have the ability to exercise 'freedom of choice' in ways that benefit themselves. The creation of conditions for self-governance is facilitated through particular forms of expertise, such as psychology, sociology, and social work, which define normal behaviour and instill the appropriate values and dispositions in people. Within the neo-liberal framework, people are seen as essentially autonomous, self-interested, competitive, and motivated solely by the desire to gain pleasure and avoid pain. This idea stands in contrast to the view that people have no intrinsic nature but become humans through the process of living in society (Tesh, 1988: 158). A key manifestation of the neo-liberal rule is the emphasis on active citizenship. The assumption that people should play an active role in managing their own affairs, for example through adopting strategies of personal risk minimization, has become as pervasive in discussions about 'the new genetics' as in other spheres of social life. One of our aims in this book is to show how the language of active citizenship, apparent in arguments for greater citizen 'participation', protection of people's 'right to choose' and 'freedom of choice', and so on, informs discussions about genetics and its benefits.

Issues of freedom of choice and public benefit have particular significance in the area of human genetics since virtually all debates take place against a background of ongoing concerns about the resurgence of eugenics, or the coercive manipulation of the human gene pool (Conrad and Gabe, 1999b: 5). Eugenics has been practised in many avowedly liberal democratic societies in the past, including the United States, the UK, and the Scandinavian countries. And a form of eugenics continues to be practised today in China, where a Eugenics Law (euphemistically called the Maternal and Infant Health Law) was passed in 1995 (Dikötter, 1998). In contemporary liberal democratic societies at least, eugenic attempts to control the human gene pool are seen to represent an unacceptable intrusion by the state into the lives of groups and individuals. For many people it is strongly associated with Orwell's vision of Big Brother, and the racial cleansing efforts of the Nazi period (Duster, 1990). The issue of eugenics keeps being raised by groups such as the disabled, homosexuals, and ethnic minorities, who have in the past been the target of attempts at eradication (Horgan, 1993; Le Vay, 1996; Newell, 1999a, 1999b, 1999c; Shakespeare, 1995, 1998, 1999a, 1999b; Zilinskas and Balint, 2001). Feminists have also expressed concern about the potential for genetic technologies to be used for sex selection and ethnic discrimination (e.g. Cassel, 1997; Katz Rothman, 1998: 199–206; Lippman, 1992, 1999; Mahowald, 1996, 1997, 2000; Mahowald *et al.*, 1996; Rothenberg and Thomson, 1994). (See Chapter 7.) Many critical commentators see the application of genetic knowledge as a political and human rights issue. Proponents of the new genetic technologies need to constantly persuade sceptics about the benefits of genetics for the individual, for improving their health and wellbeing, as well as the wellbeing of the community as a whole. Hence, proponents distinguish 'the new genetics' from the older eugenics by placing emphasis on personal empowerment, increased choice, and anticipated health benefits. In Chapter 2 we examine some of the history and contending definitions of the term 'the new genetics', how it is seen to differ from the 'old' eugenics, and how it has been used in the context of discussions about its benefits for the health of 'the public'.

In the context of the new genetics, the individual is conceived not as a passive recipient of expert advice, but as an *active* seeker of information and 'consumer' of health care services. The creation of new categories of genetically 'at risk' information seekers, decision-makers and consumers is one aspect of a broader transformation in notions of the person evident in many contemporary societies, involving an emphasis on the enterprising, responsible subject (Novas and Rose, 2000). This view of the subject is reiterated in various spheres of expert knowledge and practice, particularly in genetic counselling, which is based on the philosophy of 'non-directiveness'. (See Chapter 5.) The individual is seen as having a 'right to know' about their genetic health, so that they can make 'informed', voluntary decisions. That this premise is widespread was underlined by a thirty-six nation survey, undertaken between 1993 and 1995, which found that both patients and genetics professionals (including medical geneticists and genetic counsellors) value the patient's right to genetic services and information that would assist decision-making (Wertz, 1999). This 'triumph of autonomy' not only makes it difficult to draw lines in service provision, but also creates a market for services not offered by national health plans or managed care (Wertz, 1999: 173).

Arguments about people's right to genetic information are often couched in terms of the potential of such information to 'empower' the individual. Without appropriate information, it is argued, the individual cannot know that they are making the most appropriate choice about health and life-style. Admittedly, there is a great deal of debate among experts about the question of what constitutes appropriate information, and some concerns about whether indeed it is always in the best interests of the individual to know about their genetic health (see, for example, Chadwick *et al.*, 1997). However, the premise that information is necessarily 'empowering' for the individual health 'consumer' because it will offer them more 'choice' is, in the main, taken as a given.

Publications such as *Your Genes, Your Choices*, published by the American Association for the Advancement of Science (Baker, undated), emphasize the importance of 'genetic literacy' and 'informed choice' for democratic participation. Such publications, which are increasingly common in the area of public health and health promotion, serve a role in nurturing a new form of self-awareness in regard to genetics, risk, prevention and associated responsibilities. (See Chapter 5.) The book notes that, although 'you may feel that you have little control over the way that genetic research will be used, for good or for bad ... you do have power'.

> The way that society uses its knowledge of genetics will be shaped by the everyday choices its citizens make. You help shape what happens through the way you express your beliefs and opinions and by the actions you take. You also affect what happens through your community efforts, working for the passage of laws or electing leaders who believe as you do. You made a choice to gain some control of genetic issues by reading this book. Now you have the choice to remain informed. You have the choice to use your knowledge when making personal decisions that involve the use of genetic research. And you have the choice to participate when issues involving genetics are raised in your community.
>
> (Baker, undated: 70)

As some writers have argued, 'knowing your genes' means knowing your biological constraints and accepting a certain biologically allocated place in society (Love, 1996: 25). It means recognizing that 'we are not genetically equal' and that 'no matter how much we tinker with our genes, we never will be' (Baker, undated: 69). In the recent literature, there has been a great deal of emphasis on the effects on a person's 'sense of self' and 'individuality' of being informed about their genetic inheritance. These concerns are reflected in recent ethical debates about 'the right to know and the right not to know' (Chadwick, 1997). One's right to genetic information is seen to carry certain responsibilities – particularly to one's self, one's family, and one's future offspring. As the individual is constantly reminded, genetic inheritance binds the self to others, hence 'genes do not just provide an individual with identity, they also relate persons to one another and give them an identity as "relatives"' (Strathern, 1995: 104). One of the identified characteristics of the new genetics is its 'family focus'. (See Chapter 2.) It has long been recognized that diseases 'run in families'. However, the explanations as to why this is so have changed through time. With the emergence of the new genetics, the family has become a 'factor of risk' in the transmission of genetic disease, and hence a site for preventive intervention. Meanwhile, the broader economic and social conditions that shape people's life chances, health, and sense of wellbeing are largely ignored. As Julie Clague (1998) argues, the immediate impact of the HGP on health care will not be great since many of the serious health problems in the developed and developing worlds are not genetic in character. Rather, factors such as economic wellbeing, social class, place of birth and the availability of health services affect a person's chances of contracting disease (Clague, 1998: 11). These social 'factors of risk' tend to be submerged in discussions about the personal and familial genetic 'factors of risk'.

Risk and decision-making

In the area of genetic-based public health, as in other areas of public health, estimations of risk are considered to be crucial in the process of decision-making, in planning for, and if necessary insuring against, future eventualities (Petersen and Lupton, 1996). Thus, the individual as a rational being should weigh up all the 'pros' and 'cons' of all available options for action in light of estimations of genetic risk, and decide upon the most appropriate course of action. In genetic counselling, risk information is seen by counsellors as crucial in assisting people to make decisions about their family planning, employment choices, and the like. This assumes that information about statistical risk is unproblematic and that individual decisions are independent of the social context and unaffected by social experience – both highly dubious assumptions. Risk information tends to be communicated by experts in probability terms – as a ratio or percentage – which swathes it in an aura of science, making it appear beyond contention. It is assumed that the meaning of risk information is transparent to all potential users and that it is necessarily useful to people. As in many areas of health promotion, decision-making in relation to genetic information is seen to follow the cognitive model of psychology, whereby perceived vulnerability is perceived to be a major factor in motivating people to avoid risky behaviour and to initiate precautionary action (Joffe, 1999: 70). This psychological model denies the fact that actions are always constrained by the social context, with different contexts providing different degrees of 'autonomy' and 'freedom' to act. It disregards people's own lay understanding of risk, which is based on their life-world knowledge. When people fail to interpret risk information or change their behaviour in the ways expected by experts, this is defined as 'irrational' and indicative of a 'cognitive deficit', which is to ignore people's own understanding, their own 'logic' or 'rationality'. Experts often fail to acknowledge people's emotional response to risk information (Joffe, 1999), which can be profound, especially when it is seen to affect reproductive decisions.

In the book we seek to expose and critically examine a number of key assumptions that guide thinking about genetics and its applications in the promotion of 'the public's' health. These include the assumption that people tend to behave according to the above model of rational decision-making, and that one can make a clear conceptual separation between the individual and society, the private and the public, the subject and the object, nature and culture, and facts and values. A fundamental premise underlying our investigation is that science is unable to provide unmediated access to 'the truth' of our being; that language constitutes our reality, and guides the ordering of social and personal life. Hence, we undertake critically to analyse the language of genetics as it appears in public health discourse, including the use of dichotomies such as biology/culture, nature/nurture, individual/society, public/private, and new/old, and of terms such as 'the right to know' and 'freedom of choice'. In particular, we are interested in how the selection of particular metaphors in genetics, such as the representation metaphor (evident in the use of the word 'map') and the information metaphor (evident in the use of the word 'code'), shapes thinking and action (Hedgecoe, 1999). The choice of particular words, metaphors and analogies is always strategic, and directs thought and action along some avenues and not others. This is a fact recognized by scientists, who seek to promote the importance of their work through the media and other means in order to ensure wide support, and hence continued public funding, for their work. (See Chapter 4.) While the importance of language has as yet not been widely recognized by practitioners who work in the field of public health, we believe that the use of language is crucial for how problems are thought about and acted upon.

The 'nature'/'culture' dichotomy

Recent work in the social sciences and humanities has sought to reveal the dichotomies that underlie our descriptions of the natural and social world, and to explore the political and practical implications of our continuing adherence to these dichotomies. Although scientists have tended to posit a clear conceptual separation between 'nature', or 'biology', and 'culture', or 'society', in line with the view that self-understanding and social development involve liberating humans from the constraints of nature, it has become evident that these dichotomies have collapsed (Rheinberger, 1995: 257). As recent work has made clear, there are inextricable links between our conceptions and evaluations of nature and culture, and our views of the person and the human body. The language that we use to describe our humanness and 'sense of self' inevitably reflects views about how we believe the social and natural worlds 'normally' function, or should function. For much of the last two hundred years, society has been described as an organism, comprising functionally inter-related parts and governed by underlying law-like universal mechanisms. Many contemporary views of society first appeared in the nineteenth century during a period of rapid industrialization and social change, when physics provided the benchmark for scientific practice and the ideals of objective inquiry. 'Society' began to be seen as an object, subject to understanding in the same way as the physical world. Like nature, society was seen to have its own dynamic, and its own health and pathologies, which can be objectively understood (Rabinow, 1989: 24). An organic metaphor was evident in nineteenth century concerns about the 'diseases of civilization': the notion that the social body itself was sick. Tuberculosis was seen as a classic disease of civilization, and its incidence was associated with the big city's unwholesome environment: damp, smoke, over-crowding.

Alongside the conception of society as governed by law-like mechanisms, there has existed the view that humans are able to utilize knowledge to perfect society and gain greater self-understanding (Rabinow, 1989: 24). For example, science was utilized for the study of epidemics to understand and control the spread of disease with a view to improving individual bodies and the social body as a whole. Public health proponents frequently look back to the nineteenth century as an example of how rational knowledge of science combined with rational administration can alleviate pathologies which threaten the health of individual bodies and the social body as a whole (Petersen et al., 1999: 116–18). The will to perfect society, reflected in the strategies and practices of public health, has been underpinned by a vision of purity and order. As Bauman indicates, in his book *Postmodernity and its Discontents* (1997), the vision of purity has been a recurring theme in modern Western societies and has played a crucial role in establishing order, or putting everything in its rightful place. Purity is an ideal, a vision of the condition that is yet to be created, and hence requires constant vigilance against the dirt, the filth, and the 'polluting agents'. Thus, hygiene (that is, separating the pure from the impure) necessitates human intervention, rather than simply leaving things to chance (Bauman, 1997: 7). Hygienic measures have been targeted not only on the physical environment but also on human beings, who are often conceived of as an obstacle to the proper 'organization of environment', and thus treated as dirt, to be cleansed, or got rid of; for example, homosexuals, the disabled, the genetically impaired (Bauman, 1997: 8). Concerns about separating the pure from the impure have been clearly manifest in contagion theory, which postulates that illness is contagious. In practice, this has meant keeping sick people away from well people, particularly through quarantine. At times, it has resulted in the forceful seizure and forced confinement or execution of those who are assumed to cause the disease (Tesh, 1988: 11–16). The eugenics programmmes of the early twentieth century reflected this desire to rid the environment of impure elements, expressed most clearly in recurrent concerns about maintaining the 'purity of the blood' and efforts at 'racial cleansing' (Kevles, 1995: 46–7, 74–6).

Like society, the individual body has been viewed as governed by law-like mechanisms, as comprising functionally inter-related parts, and as being subject to control, improvement, and perfection by its 'owner' – the rational self. Both body and mind have been seen, in turn, as subject to rational understanding and control through science. Psychology emerged in the late nineteenth century as the science of the mind, while medicine developed as the science of bodily disease and its management. Early twentieth century ideas about health reflected the impact of the new science of bacteriology, which brought laboratory techniques to bear on attempts to understand the role of microorganisms in causing disease (Martin, 1994: 24). By the 1940s and 1950s, the most important threats to health were seen to lie in 'the environment' just outside the body. The body was viewed as a machine, comprising parts that were vulnerable to breakdown, particularly through attack by disease. Just as a society needs to maintain order by protecting itself from threats from 'enemies' (both from within and outside society), the body needs to establish its homeostasis and protect itself from the threats of germs and viruses. The task was seen as shielding the body from attack by paying attention to hygiene, the use of antiseptics, and improving the body's defence mechanisms (Martin, 1994: 23–32). In the twentieth century the discipline of psychology played a key role in the shaping of selves that were attuned to the task of promoting their own bodily integrity and efficiency, through engagement with practices of self-care, hygiene, self-improvement, and so on (Rose, 1989). The family, in particular, became a focus for the inculcation of medico-hygienic norms, through the regulation of its members and the socialization of offspring, without the threat of coercion and the direct intervention of political authorities into the household. As Rose explains, psychological techniques have had a crucial role in assisting families to govern their intimate relations and their children according to social norms through the activation of their individual desires, aspirations, and fears (1989: 130).

The 'selfish gene' and the 'genetic self'

Maintaining a conceptual separation between 'the body' and 'the self' is just as difficult to do, if not impossible, as doing so between 'nature' and 'culture'. Take, for example, the terms 'selfish gene' and the 'genetic self'. The idea that genes are endowed with the human characteristic of 'selfishness' was popularized by Richard Dawkins in his 1976 book *The Selfish Gene*. In the book Dawkins referred to human beings as 'survival machines – robot vehicles that are blindly programmed to preserve the selfish molecules known as genes' (Dawkins, 1976, cited in Nelkin and Lindee, 1995: 53). In line with Darwin's evolutionary vision of 'survival of the fittest', every gene – the fundamental unit of selection – will fight for itself and its own species. Genes act in competition, and only the strongest genes win (Van Dijck, 1998: 92–3). The gene is ascribed with agency, and is seen to be 'self-directive' and to act in the manner of a person, with an ego, a sense of purpose, and responsibilities. The notion that every organism exhibits some degree of aim or purpose – anticipates the future and chooses among alternative courses to adjust its own behaviour to what it expects to encounter – has been elaborated in the emergent cybernetic conception of evolution. Increasingly, 'survival' has to do with gathering information about the environment, anticipating change, and then responding appropriately. 'Self-organization', by way of negative and positive feedback, becomes as important as 'natural selection' in securing the survival of the organism and its offspring (Rifkin, 1998: 208–13).

A conception of 'the selfish gene' is elaborated, for example, by Matt Ridley in his book *Genome: The Autobiography of a Species in 23 Chapters* (1999), which presents an autobiographical account of the genome ('the complete set of human genes'). In the book Ridley describes the body as a 'vehicle for the genes, as a tool used by genes in their competition to perpetuate themselves .... The body's survival is secondary to the goal of getting another generation started.' (Ridley, 1999: 128) The image of the autonomous, 'self-directed' ego is reflected in his account of reproduction ('self assembly') – described as a 'decentralized process'. That is: 'Since every cell in the body carries a complete copy of the genome, no cell need wait for instructions from authority; every cell can act on its own information and the signals it receives from its neighbours' (1999: 175). Furthermore, as in modern bureaucratic societies, there exists a system of hierarchy, authority, and command. Thus, the controlling genes 'know when to delegate' (to lose control over their creation – i.e. the body – to allow learning and memory), and to convey instructions to 'unneeded cells [to] commit mass suicide' (to prevent cancer). Also, as is prescribed by the ideal bureaucratic chain of command: 'The dying cells obediently follow a precise protocol' (1999: 219, 232).

On the other hand, as many writers have noted, the concept of the person is increasingly defined in terms of genetic make-up – hence, the concept of the 'genetic self' (e.g. Keller, 1992; Nelkin and Lindee, 1995; Strathern, 1995). As Peters *et al.* note: 'Genetic information can be an important factor in defining self, family, and community ... DNA is most basic to the concept of who we are since our genetic makeup is unlike that of any other person except an identical twin' (1999: 8). The idea that our identities are defined by our genetic uniqueness is particularly evident in the use of 'genetic fingerprinting', which has become common since 1986, when this technology was used to solve a widely publicized British murder case. It now constitutes a powerful form of evidence in many criminal cases. Seen as a non-intrusive and uncomplicated procedure, DNA fingerprinting is gaining increasing appeal to the military, law enforcement and other governmental authorities, to gain evidence to establish the identity of a dead body, a missing person, a biological relative, or the perpetrator of a crime (Nelkin and Andrews, 1999: 191). Belief in the power of DNA to define identity would seem to represent an important shift in thinking about the role of 'nature' in 'what it means to be human' from that which prevailed in the 1950s and 1960s (Keller, 1992). In response to Nazi eugenics, many people began to make a strict distinction between 'nature' and 'nurture', with the latter, rather than the former, being seen to provide the foundation for human development. That is, genetics was confined to purely physiological attributes, while behaviour came to be seen as belonging to the domain of culture (Keller, 1992: 285–6). However, in the late 1960s the development of techniques for manipulating the 'Master Molecule' – for sequencing it, synthesizing it, and altering it – changed our historical sense of the immutability of 'nature'. The technological innovations of molecular biology lent credence to the notion that 'nature' could be more readily controlled than 'nurture' (Keller, 1992: 288). As the 'genetic world-view' (Miringoff, 1991) becomes more widespread, it is likely that more and more people will define themselves – gain their 'sense of identity' – or be defined by others according to their particular genetic make-up. As we explain in Chapter 7, responses to this development thus far have been diverse, providing the foundation for novel forms of citizenship that are profoundly affecting how we think about self and society.

New knowledge, new power

In seeking to make sense of recent developments in genetics and public health, we have found Michel Foucault's work on 'bio-power' to be invaluable. According to Foucault (1980), in modern societies power is a productive force that focuses on the biological existence of a population. Whereas in pre-modern societies power is concentrated in a single authority (the sovereign) and manifest in the right to kill, in modern societies power is diffuse and exercised over life itself (1980: 141). The task of authorities is not to impede or destroy life, but rather to sustain life and subject it to precise controls and regulations so that its capabilities are optimized. In Foucault's view, this 'power over life', or 'bio-power', evolved in two basic forms. One centres on the body as a machine, and involves its disciplining and the optimization of its capacities – what he called an 'anatomo-politics of the human body'. The other focuses on the 'species body, the body imbued with the mechanics of life and serving as the basis of the biological processes: propagation, births and mortality, the level of health, life expectancy and longevity, with all the conditions that can cause these to vary'. This latter form is supervised through 'an entire series of interventions and regulatory controls: a biopolitics of the populations' (1980: 139). Norms, particularly sexual norms, have become increasingly important for the 'management of life'. If life is to be brought within the realm of explicit calculations and made the subject of transformation and improvement, there is a need for 'continuous regulatory and corrective mechanisms'. Thus, issues of measurement, classification, and appraisal have become crucial to the operation of power. In Foucault's view, the eugenics movement, with its concerns about 'blood relations' and the purity of the 'blood line', and racism 'in its modern, "biologizing" statist form' are clear manifestations of bio-power (Foucault, 1980: 145–50).

The HGP, and other gene-mapping initiatives, symbolize the discourses and practices of bio-power. (On this point, see Rabinow, 1992.) By revealing disease and proper functioning at the molecular level, the HGP promises ultimate control over life processes. The web site 'Human Genome Project Information' notes that:

> Medical practices will be radically altered when powerful new clinical technologies based on DNA diagnostics are combined with information emerging from genome maps. Emphasis will shift from treatment of the sick to a prevention-based approach. Researchers will be able to identify individuals predisposed to particular diseases and devise novel therapeutic regimes based on new classes of drugs, immunotherapy techniques, avoidance of environmental conditions that may trigger disease, and possible replacement of defective genes through gene therapy. The ability to sequence DNA directly and quickly will revolutionize mutation research by allowing researchers to study directly the relationships between disease and exposure to various agents. Data from these studies could be coupled with medical information to diagnose disease onset and develop therapeutic strategies. ... What we learn about human genetics will help us to raise healthier, more productive, disease-resistant farm animals that might, through wise and careful genetic engineering, produce drugs of value to us.
>
> (http://www.ornl.gov/hgmis/faq/faqs1.html)

As this description makes clear, proponents of the HGP have little doubt about the potential of genomic research to alter medical practice, and to deliver benefits by way of an improved understanding, treatment and prevention of disease. The difficulties of classifying diseases, faced by every theory of medicine in human history, promise finally to be resolved by genetics (Lloyd, 1994). It is believed that diseases will be subject to precise scientific classification, analysis, and treatment. The ability to 'sequence DNA', referred to above, is seen as essential to the process of classification. Sequencing of the human genome will allow for the detailed description of the molecular causes of diseases, the comparison of 'abnormal' genes, and the development of more targeted preventive and therapeutic techniques. 'Abnormal' genes can be isolated, then altered, replaced, or simply discarded (1994: 100–1). Terms such as 'genetic abnormality' or 'genetic defect' in many descriptions of genetic technologies convey a vision of the broken body-machine, which needs to be 'corrected' or 'fixed'.

Anticipated new gene therapies

The gene therapy industry, which has burgeoned in recent years, has been founded on the premise that genetic diagnostics will find a ready market for its products. Although the development of gene therapies is in its infancy, experts predict that gene therapy will be applied to a vast range of diseases, including cancers, neuromuscular disorders, cystic fibrosis, and even polygenetic and multifactorial disorders such as hypertension and diabetes mellitus. The idea of getting to the root cause of inherited disease, by correcting faulty genes or adding healthy genes that are missing, has great appeal to scientists (Tagliaferro and Bloom, 1999: 264; see also Friedmann, 1994). Critics, however, point out that not enough is presently known about gene function to attempt gene therapy (Tagliaferro and Bloom, 1999: 267). The idea of gene therapy is highly controversial, particularly in the aftermath of the widely publicized death in 1999 of an American teenager, Jesse Gelsinger, in a gene therapy experiment that went wrong. Gene therapy experiments continue, however, and the promise of imminent 'breakthroughs' is kept alive by periodic news reports of promising research. For example, a recent article announced that scientists 'have achieved a significant breakthrough in the struggle to make gene therapy work against cancer by using a genetically engineered virus to shrink and in some cases eliminate tumours' (Meek, 2000: 9).

Until relatively recently a major impediment to the commercial development of gene therapies has been public resistance to the notion of modifying people at the molecular level. The idea of gene therapies was first proposed in the late 1950s, but it was not until the early 1990s that the social and political context was favourable to their commercial development (Martin, 1998). Firstly, it was necessary to nurture public acceptance of the idea that genetic disease could be predicted, and that the gene, as a self-replicating mechanism, was subject to 'damage' and 'repair' and could therefore be 'fixed' by future technologies (Van Dijck, 1998: 97). As Van Dijck argues, the development of diagnostic tools, marketed particularly to women, who were anxious to assure the health and normalcy of their offspring, was important in promoting the 'actuarial mindset'. Terms such as 'genetic susceptibility', 'genetic predisposition' and 'genetic tendency' emphasize the inherent risks of living and the uncertainties that are already stored in our genes (Van Dijck, 1998: 98). Secondly, it was necessary to overcome strong resistance to what had long been seen as a neo-eugenic treatment for genetic diseases (Martin, 1998). A vision of somatic cell therapy as a solution to incurable life-threatening diseases was established and used to mobilize support among scientists and the public. The incorporation of opponents' concerns about the dangers of human genetic engineering into the regulatory regime ensured that a stable network of support for gene therapies as a 'solution' for life-threatening diseases was created (Martin, 1998: 151–3).

Given concerns about the reincarnation of eugenics via the backdoor of screens, treatments, and therapies (Duster, 1990), proponents of the new genetics have sought to emphasize the personal benefits for 'consumers' of new drugs, therapies, and preventive strategies, and the 'choices' that will eventuate. The author of an article, appearing as the cover story of Time.com, notes:

> Before this century [the twentieth century], medicine consisted mainly of amputation saws, morphine and crude remedies that were about as effective as bloodletting. The flu epidemic of 1918 killed as many people (more than 20 million) in just a few months as were killed in four years of World War I. Since then, antibiotics and vaccines have allowed us to vanquish entire

classes of diseases. As a result, life expectancy in the U.S. jumped from about 47 years at the beginning of the century to 76 now. But 20th century medicine did little to increase the natural life-span of healthy humans. The next medical revolution will change that, because genetic engineering has the potential to conquer cancer, grow new blood vessels in the heart, block the growth of blood vessels in tumours, create new organs from stem cells and perhaps even reset the primeval genetic coding that causes cells to age.

(Isaacson, 1999: 1)

According to this narrative, genetic research will provide the foundation for the next revolution or 'new wave' in treatment and prevention – a story that is recounted almost daily in the print news media. (See Chapter 4.) A news article, boldly headlined 'New gene joins cancer battle', announces that: 'An international medical team has added a new tumour-suppressing gene to the potential arsenal of genetic weapons against cancer, and may have found clues about why some cancers are more aggressive than others.' It explains that physicians in the US and Italy have been able to shrink tumours in the lungs of laboratory mice by replacing damaged copies of a gene, and that: 'Genetic therapy trials already have proved effective against cancerous tumours in humans' (*The Weekend Australian*, 29–30 January, 2000: 7). Another article, 'Gene therapy for heart vessels', announces that: 'Scientists are fast developing a powerful weapon in the fight against heart disease, by discovering how some hearts grow new blood vessels to replace blocked ones.' In the article the discovery is described as having 'led to a successful early trial of a gene therapy that promotes vessel growth, and to development of a simple blood test to identify patients who are likely to be able to grow new vessels' (Hickman, 1999: 7). Such news stories lend the impression that science is an incremental process of discovering 'the facts' about the genetic basis of disease and that effective treatment or cure is just around the corner. They reflect confidence in the ability of medicine to better control, if not conquer, disease and to offer individuals new choices, or a more 'personalized medicine'. As we will explain in Chapter 4, rarely do such stories discuss polygenetic disorders or acknowledge likely non-genetic influences on the development of disease. The overall impression conveyed by such stories is that diseases are the result of a single 'defective' gene that can be 'corrected' through simple 'quick fix' medical solutions. They reinforce the view that disease and illness are fundamentally a product of individual pathology, rather than of the social or physical environment, and that the maintenance or restoration of health occurs through the purchase of goods and services available in the marketplace rather than through social change.

The logic of 'the market'

Genetic research is seen to obey the logic of 'the market', driven by the 'demand' of 'consumers' for access to knowledge and technologies that will assist them in their efforts both to avoid illness and to achieve autonomy. As is explained in a *Guardian Weekly* article, 'Human gene code deepens mystery of life', which reported the release of information on the genetic code of a representative human ('the book of humankind'), such medicine will be 'tailored' to the individual:

> Scientists who raced to complete a document so long that it may never be printed in full said the human genome could open an era of a new kind of medicine – one tailored to a patient's unique genetic makeup. 'It will be an individualised medicine where we'll treat the individual person for the right disease, with the right medicine, at the right dose, at the right time', said Mike Dexter, director of the Wellcome Trust, the charity that launched the British research.
>
> (Radford, 2001: 1)

The provision of 'over the counter' genetic testing in recent years is an example of how the assumptions and language of consumerism and individualism inform thinking about new genetic technologies. In Britain, where the direct marketing of cystic fibrosis (CF) carrier testing to the public was announced in 1994, many people have expressed concern about the implications of this development for the health and wellbeing of 'consumers' (Harper, 1997: 68). Public health experts and other commentators fear that commercial rather than 'health benefit' considerations have been paramount in the development of such testing and that 'the market' provides no comprehensive framework of information that allows fully informed consent and decision-making. Harper, for instance, has argued that direct marketing of such tests provides no guarantee that ancillary information (apart from assistance for those concerned by receiving an abnormal result) or counselling will be provided. The expansion of 'over the counter' testing for conditions such as Alzheimer's and familial breast cancer, where results have direct and serious implications for the future health of many people, and for that of relatives, raises myriad questions. These include: how do people interpret the results? Who has access to the tests? How are the interests of minors and other third parties to be safe-guarded? And, what is the affect of test results on insurance premiums? (Harper, 1997: 71)

The 'consumer' figures prominently in surveys that seek to gauge 'the public's' perceptions of 'biotechnology'. As Davison *et al.* point out, although surveys are generally taken for granted as neutral tools for investigating public attitudes, they are 'far from innocent instruments' and constitute 'important and powerful ways of constructing "publics" and shaping public discourse ...' (1997: 330). Surveys of the public understanding of science do not simply 'measure' the understandings, opinions, fears, and attitudes of 'the public', but also embody assumptions about how 'consumers' 'normally' think and act. For example, the Eurobarometer (1993) on Biotechnology, the survey conducted by the European Union in each country to sample public perceptions of modern biotech-nology, included questions which presuppose a consumerist orientation to biotechnologies (Hill and Michael, 1998: 206). Similarly, a survey conducted by the Food and Drink Federation into the desirability of labelling genetically modified foods constructed 'the public' as wanting 'clear labelling' by suggesting that 'it' will want to do its rational decision-making at the point of purchase (Hill and Michael, 1998: 210–11). As Hill and Michael argue, such surveys have often been undertaken in the context of concerns about public resistance to 'biotechnology' and thus can be seen as a way of 'engineering acceptance' of biotechnologies. Such surveys advantage particular versions of 'biotechnology', while promoting its 'acceptability' through emphasizing such aspects of the lay person as, for example, his or her autonomy and rationality (1998: 202).

The claim that 'the new genetics' will herald a new array of treat-ment and prevention options has been criticized on the grounds that the complexity of the genetic basis of common diseases will make accurate prediction difficult if not impossible (see Holtzman and Marteau, 2000). The view that drugs can be developed to treat a

genetic-related condition, as in the developing field of pharmacogenetics (see, for example, McCarthy, 2000; Sneddon, 2000), implies
that a gene or combination of genes is the sole or main factor
underlying disease. As Holtzman and Marteau point out, such
arguments deny the potentially substantial role of other non-genetic
factors, such as the environment, on the development and manifestation of disease. As they argue, the claim that genetics will
revolutionize medicine has been surrounded by 'hype', and 'differences in social structure, lifestyle, and environment account for
much larger proportions of disease than genetic differences' (2000:
143–4). Despite such criticisms of the alleged benefits of new
genetic technologies, many writers agree that genetics is likely to
radically transform the physical and social worlds through efforts to
'remake nature'. Commentators, writing from diverse viewpoints
and with different commitments, predict that genetics will vastly
extend the ability of humans to control and administer life itself. It
is believed that this control and administration of life will be
assisted by new computer technologies, which will facilitate the
collation, storage, and processing of large quantities of genetic
information. The merging of genetic and digital technologies will
create a powerful alliance, setting the scene for a genetically engineered future and radically new forms of social organization.

In his book *The Biotech Century* (1998), Jeremy Rifkin argues
that genetics will radically change the future, by allowing scientists,
corporations, and governments to control the natural world, and
'make nature' in their own image. Such control will be concentrated in the hands of these groups, while the products will be
marketed under the guise of expanding freedom of choice for
millions of consumers (Rifkin, 1998: 172). The coming together of
the information sciences and the life sciences will allow humans to
manipulate information as never before and to create virtual
biological environments from which to model complex biological
organisms, networks, and ecosystems. Computers will allow scientists to create new synthetic molecules with a few keystrokes,
thereby bypassing the tedious process of attempting to synthesize
a real molecule in a laboratory (1998: 194). Technologies such as
the DNA chip, which scientists claim will be able to scan an individual patient, read his or her genetic make-up in precise detail,
and detect abnormal or malfunctioning genes, highlight the possibilities deriving from the union of genes and computers (1998:
178–96). Aside from the development of new medicines for the

treatment of the sick, such technologies will help to lengthen the natural human life span. While the bacteriological revolution is seen as successful in terms of producing antibiotics and vaccines to control many diseases that limit people's natural term of life, genetics challenges the very concept of the natural.

As developments in human genetics and the accompanying redefinition of the concepts of the natural and the normal gain pace, some writers suggest that it will become increasingly difficult to draw the line between treatment and enhancement in medicine. The goal of medicine is often defined with reference to some hypothetical normal functioning, the assumption being that health care ought to help people become 'normal'. There is an implied contrast between medical services that *treat* disease or disability conditions and uses that merely *enhance* human performance or appearance (Parens, 1998: 4). This distinction has been used both to articulate the content of health care and to limit medicalization, by identifying 'the proper domain' of medicine. However, as Parens argues, this distinction is problematic in that it is arbitrary and overlooks the fact that both kinds of intervention are *improvements* (Parens, 1998: 5). As biotechnological developments unsettle established notions of the natural and the normal, and allow the possibility of the selection of particular traits, the goal and role of medicine will undergo radical redefinition. With the routine use of genetic tests, the quest for perfection may overshadow the effort to eliminate genetic disease.

In Rabinow's view, the new genetics is likely to be a far greater force for reshaping society than was the revolution in physics, 'because it will be embedded throughout the social fabric at the microlevel by medical practices and a variety of other discourses' (Rabinow, 1992: 241). The increasing pervasiveness of genetic ideas, and persistent efforts to model nature on culture, he believes, are likely to eventually lead to the collapse of the nature/culture dichotomy. New groups and new identities and practices will arise out of the new genetic truths, and these will provide the foundation for new forms of sociality – 'biosociality'. For example, there will be groups that meet to share their experiences, lobby for their disease, educate their children, change their home environment, and so on (1992: 244). (So-called 'genetic support groups' would seem to be an obvious example of this. See Chapter 7.) A crucial step in overcoming the nature/culture dichotomy, Rabinow explains, will be the dissolution of the modernist category of 'society', understood as an object governed by its own laws and subject to planned change. Referring to Robert Castel's (1981) analysis of 'post-disciplinary society', Rabinow sees the beginnings of the dissolution of 'society' in transformations of the concept of risk. Increasingly, direct therapeutic intervention is being replaced by, firstly, preventive strategies of social administration based on the calculation of the factors of risk and, secondly, 'the promotion of working on oneself in a continuous fashion so as to produce an efficient and adaptable subject'. According to Rabinow, the most salient aspect of this trend is the increasing institutional gap between diagnostics and therapeutics. Although this gap is not new, it is likely to widen as biosociality progresses, presenting a new range of social, ethical, and cultural problems (1992: 242).

Powers of prediction

With the capacity to precisely classify diseases, genetics is expected to provide the foundation for a new medical paradigm – predictive medicine (see, for example, Koch, 1999: 187). Utilizing developments in molecular genetics, predictive medicine combines specific knowledge of individual genetic risk and knowledge of external risk factors for the prediction and ultimate prevention of disease. As Koch notes, it implies important changes in medical practices and in the structure of medical services. This is not to say that earlier medical paradigms, so-called laboratory medicine (based on bacteriology) and preventive medicine (involving the prevention of environmental, psychological, behavioural, and lifestyle risk factors), have been totally replaced, since old paradigms continue to exist side by side and interact with the new paradigm. Rather, the proposition is that advances in molecular medicine, and consequently in genetic diagnosis, have bestowed new powers of prediction on medicine, which is transforming medical disciplines and practices that were previously unrelated to genetics. For example, cancer genetics is emerging as an important sub-speciality in the field of oncology (Koch, 1999: 189).

Again, the media represents an important site for examining beliefs about genetics and its potential – in this case its powers of prediction and prevention. For example, in a recent article in *The Australian*, 'See your own death through DNA', it is reported that:

Within 10 years, most people will be able to find out what is most likely to kill them. Their GP will take a swab of saliva or a blood sample and do a DNA test. The GP will then check the results against a list of genes behind a range of diseases, from heart disease to Alzheimer's. If the patient is lucky, by then new drugs will have been developed to treat the defect. But even if there's no cure, research suggests most people will want to know about the defect so they can plan their lifestyle, career, marriage and children to make the best of their lives. This scenario of a 'profound revolution in health' was advanced by distinguished Canadian researcher Alan Bernstein at the Canberra Press Club yesterday. He said the increasing identification of the genetic and molecular causes of disease would shift the focus of health care from treatment to prevention with the development of a generation of new drugs.

(Kerin, 2001: 3)

Scenarios such as this promise ultimate control over disease, and hence over life planning. The assumption is that such information will necessarily be 'empowering' for 'consumers', and that they will 'want to know'. Further, the reference to GPs undertaking DNA testing reflects the belief, expressed in the professional literature, that primary care is likely to take an increasingly central role in identifying genetic disease and in assisting patients to understand the implications of genetic data. (See Chapter 5.) The development of 'disease registries' and the use of patient-based longitudinal health records in general practice, described below, is based on the premise that more knowledge will enhance predictability and, ultimately, controllability (the ability to plan).

These developments are expected to affect the field of public health, too, where an understanding of gene–environment interactions is seen to present new strategies of prevention. (See Chapter 2.) Public health practitioners seem increasingly to recognize the need to integrate genetic research, policy, and programme development into their daily work and into all the sub-fields that make up public health practice. Many of the contributors to the recently published text *Genetics and Public Health in the 21st Century: Using Genetic Information to Improve Health and Prevent Disease*, for example, make a plea to incorporate genetics into areas such as environmental and occupational health, nutrition, and infectious disease control (Khoury *et al.*, 2000).

Growing recognition of the importance of the *interaction* of 'nature' and 'nurture' on population health status has underpinned the rapid development, since the mid-1980s, of the discipline of genetic epidemiology. Stimulated by advances in molecular biology, techniques of statistical modelling, and computer technology, genetic epidemiology seeks to describe and explain the distribution of genetic traits and diseases in populations or families. It is recognized that much genetic variation may go unrecognized and remain relatively innocuous unless the individual is exposed to some critical environmental agent. The range of possible environmental agents identified by genetic epidemiologists is vast, and seemingly unlimited, including such things as drugs, diet, chemicals, viruses, relationships, being of maternal age, and stress (Austin and Peyser, 2000; Dorman and Mattison, 2000). It is argued that the genetic make-up of some individuals makes them 'susceptible' to certain environments. Such individuals have been described as having 'susceptibility genes'. In occupational and environmental health, 'biomarkers' have been used to investigate the molecular mechanisms of exposure, response, and susceptibility for many common chronic diseases (Brandt-Rauf and Brandt-Rauf, 1997; Samet and Bailey, 1997).

Gene therapies are seen to offer one path to prevention by making those who are predisposed to disease less susceptible. However, in the absence of therapies, the focus remains firmly on the behaviour of those who are susceptible, and the environments that generate risks. Environmental protection strategies that have been proposed so far include a reduction in exposures in the workplace and in the home, and the supplementation of food or water with certain essential nutrients (Khoury, 1996: 1720; Zimmern, 1999: 137). One optimistic suggestion is that, in the future, environments may be tailored to the needs of subgroups with particular genetic characteristics so as to maximize their physical or cognitive development. While this may not constitute a genetic intervention as ordinarily understood, it is nevertheless an intervention based on knowledge of how genes work in various environments (Buchanan *et al.*, 2000: 8–9).

Because the workplace is seen to present a particular risk, resulting from the production of toxins, it is not surprising that new genetics technologies have found increasing application in this area. Firstly, molecular 'biomarkers' have been used to study the effect of occupational exposures and their relation to the development of chronic diseases, particularly cancer. It is believed that, because many 'biomarkers' represent a point on the causal pathway to disease, they are likely to have high predictive value. However, in the absence of appropriate treatment or preventive intervention, concerns have been raised about the uses of the resulting information; for example, discrimination, and breaches of privacy and confidentiality (Brandt-Rauf and Brandt-Rauf, 1997: 191–3). Secondly, in the US at least, technologies for detecting genetic traits and abnormalities in individuals that may have resulted from chemical exposure have been used to assist employers in hiring and placement decisions, and in deciding whether to reduce exposure to harmful chemicals. Although testing is most common in the chemical industry – for example, DuPont has included genetic screening in the regular blood and urine tests it gives job applicants and employees – it also occurs in the oil, automobile, steel, textile, electronics, and pharmaceutical industries (E. Draper, 1991: 13–14). Such susceptibility policies locate risk in the workers themselves, while diverting attention from the hazardous conditions resulting from the organization of work (1991: 177).

Genetic surveillance

With its broad focus on 'the population' and 'the family' as sites for the analysis of genetic variation and risk and for preventive intervention, genetic epidemiology presents enhanced opportunities for medical and public health surveillance. Epidemiologists and geneticists share an interest in keeping records of individuals with specific diseases for the purposes of health-care delivery, resource allocation and research. 'Disease registries', and more specifically 'birth defect registries', are seen as useful for monitoring the occurrence of various conditions that serve as early warning signals for possible detrimental effects of environmental factors. Although the avowed intention of these registries is to benefit patients who have tested positive to a genetic disorder, some registries include information about other family members, and so may be used to contact relatives who do not know they are at risk (British Medical Association, 1998: 142–50). The pressure to expand the use of such registries, and hence the collection and storage of a growing amount of personal information, is likely to increase as more and more genetic-epidemiological research is undertaken. As a consequence of the need to analyse both genetic and environmental factors simultaneously, and the interaction between them, the size of population samples in studies may be substantial. In the UK, for instance, a proposal by the Wellcome Trust and the Medical Research Council (MRC) to undertake prospective studies of genetic and environmental risk factors in later life, discussed at an expert workshop in May 1999, was anticipated to involve a sample of up to 500,000 individuals. Each of these was to be linked to personal medical records (Martin and Kaye, 2000: 175).

The potential for genetic surveillance is enhanced with the health care system's move towards patient-based longitudinal health records. In Australia, in 2000, state and federal health ministers approved a $440 million, 10-year plan to issue ID numbers linked to electronically stored personal records (Mitchell, 2000: 33). These electronic records contain all data relevant to the individual's health over a lifetime. What is foreseen is a single record for each individual, continually expanded from pre-birth to death and accessible to a wide range of individuals and institutions. It is suggested that genetic testing and screening information are likely to become an important part of longitudinal records. The principal forms include foetal (prenatal), newborn, carrier, and clinical (primary care) screening (Gostin, 1995: 321). Recently, concerns have been expressed about the storage of genetic information in 'DNA data banks', maintained with individual identifiers and in computerized form, for forensic and other purposes. In the UK the use of DNA banks has been the subject of a recent House of Lords Select Committee investigation and Human Genetics Commission (HGC) working group inquiry. (See Human Genetics Commission, undated.) International anxiety about the implications of DNA databases has been heightened in particular by the legislation from December 1998 in Iceland authorizing the creation and operation of a centralized health sector database for the whole population. (See Chapter 6.) The initiation of the database by a commercial firm, with a monopoly on the use of the information for commercial purposes, has given rise to a range of concerns, including informed consent, scientific openness, and commercial profiteering from the collective property of a whole nation (Nielsen, 1999). The idea of DNA databases for forensic purposes at least has gained widespread currency. For example, the UK, France, Germany, the Netherlands, Austria, Switzerland, the US, Canada, and Australia all operate DNA databases of similar construction and, in Europe, there is a trend towards cooperation and standardization. The UK

National DNA Database, established in 1995, was the first of its kind in the world and is rapidly increasing its sample rate (around 6,000 per week); it is expected to eventually include samples and profiles of one third of the UK male population (Human Genetics Commission, undated: 46–8). It is suggested that the DNA profile can only be used for the identification of individuals and will not ('as far as is known') provide data on genetic disorders or susceptibilities (Human Genetics Commission, undated: 45). However, the MRC/Wellcome Trust proposal, mentioned above, indicates that the notion of using genetic databases for the 'risk profiling' of the population has support among at least some sections of the medical establishment.

Bogard (1996) sees genetic technologies as fundamental to an increasingly prevalent form of surveillance, namely simulated surveillance, involving the categorization or 'profiling' of populations according to level of risk. In simulated surveillance, the gap between virtual and actual control disappears: nothing is left to chance; everything is visible in advance and subject to prediction and 'control before the event'. Simulated surveillance is facilitated through modern electronics and communications technologies, which allow for the storing and deciphering of huge quantities of genetic data and the construction of diagnostic profiles. Computers allow individuals who share certain traits or sets of traits to be grouped together in a way that decontextualizes them from their social environment and permits the objective analysis of risk factors (Rabinow, 1992: 243). Following Latour (1986), computers serve as 'inscription devices', or means by which biological information can be translated into forms which can be easily read, interpreted and reconfigured. Because location has less meaning in an electronic world, surveillance can be exercised over entire populations and families from multiple sites and remote locations. Further, with the development of profiling, surveillance no longer needs to rely on an 'external' surveillor, since the individual can compare him- or herself to the profile. That is, the individual participates in and becomes responsible for their own observation (i.e. self-surveillance) (Bogard, 1996: 28).

In recent years, there has been a growing emphasis on 'genetic literacy', that is the need for individuals to be aware of their own genetic risk and how such risk can be best minimized or managed. This emphasis is reflected in, among other sources, 'popular' health advice literature. For example, the book *Genetic Nutrition* combines nutrition advice with information from the field of genetics, and describes how to design a diet based on the medical history of one's family (Simopolous *et al.*, 1993: xi). Although, as is pointed out, one is genetically unique, one's risk is determined by one's membership of the family and ethnic group:

> Just as we do not take each other's medicines, we do not all benefit from the same diet. The reason is, pure and simple, genetics. We are each unique, made so by our individual inheritance, the myriad genes found on our forty-six chromosomes. This book will show you how to understand what your particular genetic blueprint can tell you about what you should eat. It will explain why, as a nation, we must move away from the universal public health approach, with its collective recommendations for the entire population, to a more selective, informed process that will take into account individual genetic differences in how we absorb and metabolize nutrients and how we expend energy. Now, to avoid any additional confusion right at the start, we must point out that while we are genetically unique, we got that way by mixing the genes of our biological parents. That explains what we all can see without any scientific training – families that are prone to certain conditions, such as cancer or heart disease. It also explains the genetic diseases that are found in larger numbers in one ethnic group and not another, such as cystic fibrosis in whites and sickle cell anemia in blacks and Asians. In this book, therefore, we will show you how to know your genetic self as an individual, as part of a family, and as a member of a clan.
>
> (Simopolous et al., 1993: xii)

In drawing attention to the regulatory and surveillance potential of the new genetic technologies as they are applied to advancing the public's health, we do not wish to present an overly pessimistic or overly speculative view of the potential of genetics. Fears and fantasies about genetic possibilities abound, and we would not wish to fuel them further. Our aim is to highlight how new genetic technologies – particularly as they converge with digital technologies – are shaping ways of thinking about the body, the self, and society, and to question some prevailing assumptions about the applications of new genetics and its benefits. In our view, it is timely to explore the sociocultural, politico-economic and global contexts that are shaping the uptake of genetic ideas, and to assess the implications of the strategies and practices that have been adopted or proposed thus far. Stories of new genetic 'breakthroughs' tend to be presented in the media and in science as stories of optimism and promise, and greeted by lay publics with a mixture of fascination and fear. It is our belief that there is a need for a novel perspective on the new genetics as applied to public health that recognizes its potential to profoundly transform our concepts of self and our awareness of ourselves as embodied beings. It is in its potential to alter our view of ourselves and of our relationships with others that the new genetics has its most potent effects as a form of governance. We expect that many readers will not share our predictions and conclusions about the manifestations and impacts of the new genetics. However, if our book stimulates debate and further research, we believe it will have served its purpose.

Plan of the book

The broad perspective of the book, and the areas that needed to be covered, were decided jointly. However, each of us is responsible for different chapters, with their content reflecting our own particular interests and views. In addition to this chapter, Alan Petersen wrote Chapters 2, 4, 5, and 7, while Robin Bunton wrote Chapters 3 and 6.

Chapter 2 examines the scope and context of 'the new genetics': its aims and characteristics and purported contributions to advancing 'the public's' health; its differences from, and similarities to, eugenics, and the politico-economic conditions shaping its emergence. As is argued, 'the new genetics' is often left undefined but, when defined, the ideal of 'empowerment' is highlighted, which provides a frequent point of contrast with eugenics, which is characterized and dismissed as coercive and 'pseudo-scientific'. However, recent histories that reveal the diversity of eugenic discourses and programmes complicate this characterization. The chapter explores points of convergence between the new genetics and eugenics in their broad goals, and the similar contexts giving rise to both. It investigates the integration of genetic ideas in public health at international, regional, and local levels, in a milieu of an increasingly liberalized, global market, and identifies new citizen rights and duties implied by the management of genetic risk. It points to the potential for eugenic-like outcomes arising through the collective actions of individuals exercising their rights. In conclusion, questions are raised about the implications of these developments in light of the social structural and global-level solutions that are urgently needed to reduce inequalities in health and wellbeing.

Chapter 3 examines genetic technologies as an aspect of technological change that is transforming our ways of seeing and living, and the implications of new genetic technologies for conceptions of public health. Recent critical work in science and technology studies has underpinned the visions, social relationships and networks underlying science and technology in general. New technologies, such as genetic technologies, reflect, reinforce and introduce particular social arrangements, new forms of governance. The introduction of gene therapies, for instance, sets in place a set of social relations, a particular world view, and a way of responding to health problems that seem natural and uncontestable. The chapter illustrates these points by reference to the field of public health. Although definitions of public health seem elusive and variable across contexts, common elements tend to include the triumvirate of the individual (or host), the environment (or context) and the agent (or contagion). The chapter evaluates the emerging impact of new genetic technologies on the underlying concepts of public health and highlights the broader implications for notions of society and the demarcation of the public and the private.

Chapter 4 focuses on news media portrayals of the new genetics and its applications in the advancement of 'the public's' health. The uptake of genetic ideas in medicine and public health is occurring during a period in which a burgeoning number of stories on new genetic 'breakthroughs' are appearing in the media, linked to various 'gene-mapping' initiatives, such as the HGP. The chapter investigates the media's role in portraying science and technology in general, and the relationship between scientists and the media, and presents a summary of the findings of an Australian study undertaken by one of us (AP) examining newspaper portrayals of genetics and medicine. It is argued that, while simplistic views of 'media effects' should be eschewed, by 'framing' issues as they do – selectively presenting some themes, facts and claims, and not others – the media is likely to exert a powerful influence on public definitions of genetics and its applications in treatment and prevention. The reported study confirms other research that shows that the news media tend to present a generally positive image of genetics, and shows that there is rarely mention of the influence of non-genetic influences and 'multifactorial' interactions on disorders, or questioning of the goals, direction, methods, or value of research. Such reporting is likely to offer a powerful constraint on public discourse about the new genetics and its benefits and risks.

Chapter 5 explores genetic counselling as a key site where assumptions about the empowering potential of the new genetics are articulated. Genetic counselling is expected to play an increasingly important role at the interface between scientists and lay publics, in facilitating autonomous decision-making. However, as information about genetic disease and its management becomes more widespread, the issues dealt with in genetic counselling are likely to become commonplace in other professional domains, particularly primary health care and medical practice. Given their ongoing relationship with patients/'clients' and their families, GPs are perceived as being ideally positioned to assist people in reaching 'informed' decisions. An analysis of the discourse and practices of genetic counselling, therefore, provides insights into broader processes at work in social responses to genetic disorders. The chapter outlines the historical context shaping concern with the provision and extension of counselling services, and critically examines key assumptions and characteristics of the so-called 'non-directive' approach that is widely seen as a defining feature of contemporary genetic counselling. It identifies a range of constraints on the realization of 'non-directiveness' and, in conclusion, draws attention to some of the unexamined regulatory and exclusionary implications of this implicitly consumerist approach to health.

Chapter 6 places the development of new genetic technologies in an international context, linking their development to global economic processes that can have a profound effect on health and health care. The new genetics reflects a belief in the biomedical 'quick fix' and reinforces the perspective of the so-called developed world. Although global inequalities in the distribution of communicable diseases persist, a convergence of disease patterns between 'developed' and 'developing' countries underlines the increasingly interconnected nature of the world, expressed in the term 'globalization'. Western dominance, or 'biocolonialism', is manifest in the operations of patenting and the commodification of genes, clearly evident in the Human Genome Diversity Project. The chapter examines resistance to this commodification of nature and the body, and then explores some implications of the exportation of Western cultural values via imposed technologies, examining the particular case of GM food or GMOs (genetically modified organisms). Study of 'the new genetics' and health has not usually considered the broader implications of the new genetic technologies in this context, even though the implications of biotechnology for inequalities in health have been noted. GMOs are seen to hold great promise for both profit and environmental improvement, and possibly health. As such, they are likely to be the focus of future efforts to advance the health of 'the public'. The chapter examines the implications of these globalizing processes of commodification for indigenous economies, farmers, and the environment.

Finally, Chapter 7 examines the responses of some of those groups that have been directly affected by new genetic technologies, and evaluates efforts thus far to involve 'the public' in decisions about these technologies. The chapter elaborates on some points about 'freedom of choice' and active citizenship raised in earlier chapters. With increasing attention to 'genetic literacy', and the rapid integration of genetic technologies in strategies of prevention, a growing number of people have been identified, or identify themselves, as being 'at risk' or victims of a genetic disease or disability. Many such groups have consequently organized in various ways to advance or protect their rights as citizens. While some groups have supported genetic research, and have worked closely with professionals to advance their goals, other groups, including feminists and disability rights activists and scholars, have expressed concerns about the potential of the new technologies to erode existing rights. In conclusion, the chapter recommends some caution in relation to the ideal of active citizenship, which, it is argued, is open to easy appropriation by groups with different agendas, and calls for a critical evaluation of guiding concepts and political responses and strategies in relation to new genetic technologies. The aim of the book has not been to suggest how people *should* respond to these technologies, but rather to identify some of the governing discourses surrounding 'the new genetics' as it is applied to advancing the health of 'the public', with the aim of stimulating further debate and research.

It is difficult to conclude a book of this nature, and we do not seek to offer firm conclusions here. The field of genetics and health is changing extremely quickly, making its analysis challenging and exciting. The field of study is an open one and defies singular or exclusive disciplinary perspectives. Claims of a scientific revolution of Copernican proportions carry with them myths of progress and make the adoption of these newer technologies appear 'rational' and 'inevitable'. We have argued against such a view of genetics and health. Investment in research and product development is considerable, however, and new forms of practice are being developed. Biotechnology financial markets remain vibrant (if often somewhat turbulent) and the marriage between science and industry appears to be secure. There are many emerging forms of resistance to the newer products and techniques and active political struggles. Political and moral debate is taking place in a range of settings and within many social networks. The current state of development in the field limits the possibilities for prediction. Here we have attempted to plot some emerging social patterns and issues and provide some synthesis of and commentary on topics relating to 'the public's health' and to broader changes in health care. We invite you to join us in the effort to develop new perspectives on this open and rapidly changing field, which will, no doubt, be transformed in ways that will exceed the analyses and scope of this book.

Chapter 2

The scope and context of the new genetics

Alan Petersen

This chapter explores the scope and context of the new genetics. Firstly, it describes the espoused aims and characteristics of the new genetics and its purported contributions to advancing health, and critically examines the claim that the new genetics is fundamentally different from, and opposed to, the old eugenics. It then examines the conditions shaping the emergence and application of genetic ideas in pursuit of 'the public's' health, and the manifestations of, and imperatives surrounding, the effort to manage genetic risk. In the last chapter, we began to develop our perspective on the new genetics as it is being applied in the advancement of the public's health, showing how it is changing the ways we think about the self, the body, and society. As we argued, genetic ideas are transforming the conception of public health, generating new domains for analysis and intervention, and expanding the scope of public health to include analysis of gene–environment interactions in the etiology of disease. We noted the emergence of disciplines such as genetic epidemiology, and the forms of surveillance to which this gives rise, such as birth defect registries, and how such surveillance may be facilitated by the electronic storage of information on health and the development of DNA data banks. As we mentioned, discussions about the new genetics occur against the background of persistent concerns about resurgent eugenics. Consequently, proponents take great pains to distance the new genetics from the earlier eugenics, and to emphasize its benefits for the individual and the population as a whole. It seems appropriate then to begin the chapter by examining how the new genetics has been defined and what its contributions are seen to be, before moving on to examine how it is being taken up and applied in pursuit of the public's health.

How has 'the new genetics' been defined?

The first point to note is that, like many widely used terms, 'the new genetics' is a contested term, which has been defined in various ways. Different writers identify different distinguishing elements, according to their own particular political and practical purposes. However, more often than not its meaning is left undefined by those who use it, as though its meaning is transparent and generally agreed upon, and therefore not requiring elaboration. Even in books where 'the new genetics' appears in the title, authors often fail to define the term (see, for example, Conrad and Gabe, 1999a; Gert *et al.*, 1996; Jaroff, 1991; Kidd and Kidd, 1999; Nippert *et al.*, 1999). When definitions are given, 'the new genetics' is sometimes described in terms of a distinct body of knowledge and related practices (or 'procedures'), but more frequently in relation to its ideals or aims and its expected outcomes or implications. The new genetics is seen to embody a unique set of ideals, which are regarded as best realized through particular 'enabling' practices. We shall examine some recent definitions and accounts of 'the new genetics' in order to highlight what have been identified as its distinguishing features.

According to Finkler (2000), who is an anthropologist with a research interest in genetics and kinship,

> The new genetics refers to knowledge and procedures based on DNA technology; it brings into the forefront of people's consciousness the genes carried by individuals and their families. It anticipates that by seeking testing, people will develop control over genetically inherited diseases. By doing so they might be enabled to plan their lives to the point of opting to bear only healthy children with predetermined characteristics.
>
> (Finkler, 2000: 50)

This definition draws attention to the impact of genetic ideas on people's thinking and future actions. As mentioned in the last chapter, in recent years there has been increasing emphasis on the need for people to become aware of the role of genetics in health; that is, to increase their 'genetic literacy'. The notion of the 'genetic self' emphasizes the impact of genetic ideas on one's concept of self, or identity – ideas about one's biological makeup, and ideas that may inform action (i.e. 'plan[ning] their lives'). New genetic knowledge has been promoted on the assumption that it will 'empower'

people by giving them more choice, particularly in relation to reproductive decision-making. The utilization of genetic knowledge to
enhance 'freedom of choice' in reproduction is seen by many new
genetics adherents as one of the major features of the new genetics,
distinguishing it from the old eugenics, which, it is argued, involved
infringement of many individuals' reproductive freedom. (See, for
example, Buchanan *et al.*, 2000: chapters 2, 6.)

Finkler goes on to discuss the productive power of the new
genetics. That is, genetic knowledge delineates new categories of
people and new conditions that require intervention. It is 'redrawing
the boundaries between healthy and unhealthy people because,
potentially, we are all unhealthy, or possible carriers of malfunctioning genes', and it 'reveals asymptomatic conditions that may
remain forever asymptomatic, as well as susceptibilities or risks for
developing common diseases such as breast cancer or diabetes'.
Furthermore, 'with the new genetics, the true patient becomes the
entire family rather than the individual, since to treat the individual
the family's medical history and genetic map must also be known'
(Finkler, 2000: 50). The focus on 'the family' is strongly evident in
the recent literature on public health genetics, as we note below, and
is a feature that is seen by some writers to also distinguish the new
genetics from the old eugenics, which focuses on 'the population'.
Because genes are inherited, 'the family' is affected by any decision-
making in relation to genetic health. The new genetics is seen as
having a preventive goal: by helping to identify those who are likely
to become ill, new genetic knowledge promises to point the way to
the development of novel preventive interventions. Since everyone is
potentially 'at risk' of developing a genetic disease (becoming
'unhealthy') or being a carrier of a genetic disorder, a major task is
to identify those who are 'at increased risk' for early intervention.
As one commentator observes, in the new genetics, genetic variation
becomes another form of 'risk factor' that needs to be identified
and managed (Bell, 1998).

In a recent textbook, *Practical Genetics for Primary Care*, edited
by a general practitioner and a consultant in clinical genetics, 'the
new genetics' is defined simply as 'the application of developments
in molecular biology to the study of genetics' (Rose and Lucassen,
1999). This tells us nothing about the applications of genetic ideas
in treatment or prevention, or its implications for social organization. However, the authors offer some insights into the motivations
that underlie the coining of the term 'the new genetics':

The term was first coined in 1979 to raise people's awareness of the possibility of mapping and defining the structure of genes on a scale that had not previously been possible. Prior to this, genetics had largely been confined to the study of rare diseases but advances in the laboratory opened up the possibility of studying and identifying the genetics of more common diseases as well as performing much more rapid and large scale analyses. Predictions were made that the new genetics would make a considerable impact on clinical medicine – it would lead to a better understanding of the aetiology and pathophysiology of many diseases and it could lead to a new basis on which to define diseases or a new taxonomy of disease. While genetics had previously been a rather academic branch of medicine with little intervention possible, it was predicted that these new developments could give us new diagnostic tests, options for prevention, and even new treatments. Twenty years later, these ideas are no longer 'new' and indeed they are beginning to be realized. Articles appear in the media almost daily about advances in genetic knowledge and it cannot have escaped many people's notice – health professionals as well as patients – that genetics now plays a significant role in medicine.

(Rose and Lucassen, 1999: 1)

Although one might take issue with the date of origin of 'the new genetics' specified here – we have found a somewhat earlier reference to the term (Hamilton, 1972) – commentators generally agree that the term is a relatively recent 'invention'. Again, mention is made of the issue of awareness raising in relation to the possibilities presented by genetic knowledge, for the study and identification of the genetic basis of disease, for 'performing much more rapid and large scale analyses', and for medical practice, including diagnosis, treatment, and prevention. The assumed implication of the focus on the genetics of 'common diseases' rather than 'rare diseases' is that it will have broad public benefit. However, while the authors affirm that 'genetics now plays a significant role in medicine', they provide few details about the ways in which 'the new genetics' is being, or might be, applied in treatment and prevention. Like much of the professional literature in this area, although 'the new genetics' is assumed to bring benefits, few details are provided about what the new genetics means in actual practice. However, as we will argue, many debates about the supposed benefits or dangers of the new genetics concern the very question of how the ideas are being, or are likely to be, translated into practice. For many professionals working in the area of the new genetics, a sharp distinction is often drawn between the 'new' genetics and the 'old' eugenics.

The 'new'/'old' dichotomy: professionals' use of rhetorical strategies

In a recent UK study, professional scientists and clinicians working in the area of the new genetics were found to make great efforts to distinguish between the new genetics and eugenics (Kerr *et al.*, 1998c). Eugenics was characterized as politically distorted bad science, existing in totalitarian regimes, involving the abuse of neutral scientific knowledge and having technically unfeasible aims. In contrast, the new genetics was presented as neutral scientific knowledge and technology, which is beneficial in alleviating genetic disease. As these researchers argue, experts use rhetorical strategies to distance the new genetics from eugenics, by emphasizing its offering of individual choice as opposed to societal compulsion, its 'correct' scientific basis, and its focus on the individual disease rather than the population gene pool (1998c: 177–8). In her US study of prenatal diagnosis, Rapp also found that most of the geneticists and genetic counsellors with whom she spoke 'cod[ed] the current context as one that promotes individual reproductive choice, stressing its difference from state-mandated reproductive limitations' (Rapp, 1999: 37). Implicitly or explicitly, the new genetics is often portrayed as *opposed* to the 'old' eugenics. However, like the new genetics, eugenics is often left undefined or is characterized in only the broadest of terms.

As Paul notes, in a recent critical review of the meanings of eugenics: ' "Eugenics" is a word with nasty connotations but an indeterminate meaning' and 'often reveals more about its user's attitudes than it does about the policies, practices, intentions, or consequences labeled' (1994: 143). One major source of confusion in discussions arises from the fact that some writers focus only on *intentions* while others describe *effects*. Thus, from the latter's point of view, it makes sense to call the practice of abortion following prenatal sceening 'eugenics', while from the former's it does not. As Paul explains:

Few if any women choose abortion with the aim of improving the gene pool. However, private decisions may, taken collectively, have population effects. These consequences would appropriately be labeled eugenic (or perhaps dysgenic) given some definitions – and equally inappropriate given others. And that is but one source of confusion.

(Paul, 1994: 144)

As Paul argues, it seems that what people object to in eugenics is not the goal, such as improving the health of the population, but rather the means employed to achieve it. From this perspective, where no coercion exists (e.g. law or obvious forms of social pressure), policies oriented to the good of the population are not properly labelled 'eugenic' (1994: 145).

In the liberal democratic context, 'eugenics' evokes strong reactions because it is associated with coercive control by the state or some other external authority over personal reproductive decisions. It is seen to represent an intrusion by the state on individual freedoms, which are seen as sacrosanct. For proponents of the new genetics, the word 'new' acts as a boundary marker, delineating that which promotes individual 'freedom of choice' (and is therefore assumed to be necessarily 'good') from that which denotes coercive control and lack of individual choice (and is therefore deemed 'bad'). This suggests that there is general agreement on the meaning of 'freedom of choice' and of 'coercion', which does not in fact exist. As Paul (1994) argues, although there is broad acknowledgement that coercion is bad, there is lack of agreement on what coercion *is*. Different political traditions define coercion and freedom in different ways. For classical liberals, and contemporary (libertarian) conservatives, a decision is voluntary if there are no formal, legal barriers to choice. For socialists and some other liberals, freedom to choose involves more than the removal of legal barriers; it occurs only when there is the practical ability to agree or refuse to do something. Thus, not just law but also economics can constrain choice (1994: 146). Proponents of the new genetics rarely acknowledge these complexities, however. It is simply assumed that there is general agreement on the meaning of 'freedom of choice', and that information itself is the sole necessary condition to achieve it. (For elaboration on the politics of 'freeedom of choice', see chapter 7.)

Unlike eugenics, which is focused on some members of the population with the aim of eliminating 'undesirables' (negative eugenics) or breeding of the fit (positive eugenics), the new genetics is seen to present positive options and to allow individuals to make their own 'informed' voluntary decisions. This is facilitated through 'non-directive' genetic counselling, which is frequently presented as the hallmark of the new genetics. (See Chapter 5.) A distinction is also often made in terms of period: eugenics was espoused and practised from approximately 1870 to 1950, according to many histories, whereas the new genetics emerged only in the 1980s. Accounts sometimes portray a linear progression in ideas, with objective, rational science leading the way. The new genetics is seen as based on the findings of 'disinterested' or value-neutral enquiry, whereas eugenics is seen as politically motivated 'pseudo-science'. Developments in molecular biology in the 1970s, involving the discovery and manipulation of recombinant DNA, are seen to have laid the foundation for the new genetic era, characterized by genetic diagnostics and counselling. The earlier eugenics era is often seen to involve a crude or incorrect understanding of the mechanisms of inheritance, and to be single-mindedly focused on 'nature' as the cause of human failings. While in some accounts sharp lines are drawn between the earlier eugenics period and the period of the new genetics, in other accounts the boundary is less clearly drawn, and there are seen to be some continuities, with the latter owing its origins to the former.

Although a vision of eugenics, based on various combinations of the above elements, looms large in virtually all discussions about the new genetics, recent historical scholarship suggests that the early eugenics movement was far more complex and diverse than has been depicted by many writers. This work indicates that a number of the above distinctions are less clear than has been portrayed, thereby casting doubt on proponents' accounts of the new genetics. While this is not the place to examine this work in detail, since that has already been done elsewhere, we wish to draw attention to a number of key findings, since they have implications for how one thinks about and evaluates the new genetics and its applications. They emphasize the extent to which the above dualistic distinctions have operated as a governing discourse, framing and limiting debates and influencing policies and their evaluation. The positive portrayal of the new genetics, which has served to legitimize the applications of genetics in public health, has relied upon the maintenance of a distinction between the 'new' genetics and the 'old' eugenics. In a context of widespread concerns about the implications of new genetic technologies, expressed through the media and other public forums, new genetics proponents have sought to emphasize the benefits of genetic technologies – their contributions to advancing the health and choice of individuals. Recent historical work, however, leads us to look more closely at some of the claims that have been made.

The diversity of the forms of eugenics

Buchanan *et al.* (2000) have shown that eugenics has taken many forms, varying considerably from country to country and within each nation's movement in terms of biases, beliefs about the mechanisms of transmission of inherited traits and about appropriate research and methods. The French and Brazilian eugenics movements, for example, were at least as concerned with neonatal care as with heredity, and their hereditary thinking was Lamarckian in that they believed that parents passed on to their children characteristics that were acquired during their lives. Such evidence challenges the perception, held by many contemporary commentators, that eugenics was a movement that emphasized nature over nurture as both cause and remedy of human failings (2000: 32). As Buchanan *et al.* note, although eugenicists may have shared broadly similar goals, they varied considerably in terms of their political belief, use of science, practical proposals, and legislative aims. Eugenic thinking was compatible with varied political viewpoints, being promoted by social democrats in the Nordic countries and Canada, the Fabian Socialists in the United Kingdom, the Progressives in the United States, and the Nazis in Germany. Some countries, such as the United States, Denmark and Germany, enacted involuntary sterilization legislation, while in others, such as England, involuntary sterilization was rare. Furthermore, not all eugenicists were classist or racist, or pursued eugenics goals without concern for social reform. The generation of what Daniel Kevles (1995) calls 'reform eugenicists' included those on the left who sought to develop a genetics which would be allied with medicine, freed of racial and class biases. The reformers recognized that social conditions could just as easily as heredity account for the lack of achievement of, and physical and mental disease among, lower-income groups. They argued the importance, to both eugenics and social welfare, of adequate diet, health care, housing, and education, and called for the abolition of slums, the creation of decent housing and of recreational and day-care centres, and the right to a job and a fair wage (Kevles, 1995: 173–6).

Despite the claims of many contemporary commentators, not all eugenicists believed that reproduction should be controlled by the state. Some, such as Galton, who is credited with having been the founder of eugenics, the science of 'the improvement of the human race by better breeding', hoped to secure voluntary acquiescence with eugenic guidelines by making eugenics a civil religion (Buchanan *et al.*, 2000: 42). His vision was promoted by the Eugenic Society in the UK (founded by Galton), which produced a film that sought to educate people to see their reproductive behaviour as a part of their civic responsibilities. The film encouraged viewers to examine their pedigrees and calculate their own family's fitness for marriage (Thom and Jennings, 1999: 218). Many eugenicists stressed the voluntary character of their proposals, especially in Britain where the socialist Havelock Ellis argued that 'the only compulsion we can apply in eugenics is the compulsion that comes from within' (Paul, 1994: 145). This focus on voluntary behaviour was consistent with the raison d'être of eugenics; namely that individual desire should be sacrificed for the public good (Paul, 1994: 149).

Finally, the claim that eugenics was 'bad science' or 'pseudo-science' denies scientists' contributions to eugenic thought, including their use of statistical and quantitative methods, which in the UK were promoted by Galton himself, who was a mathematician, and continued by Karl Pearson. Like contemporary genetics, eugenics was taught at leading universities, was the topic of professional science journals, and received attention in standard biology textbooks (Buchanan *et al.*, 2000: 31; Kevles, 1995: 26–40). Of course, like any science, the science of eugenics was not free of values and biases. However, to suggest that it was 'pseudo-science' implies that the new genetics is 'real' science and thus value-free. It is also important to recognize that, as with the new genetics, scientists themselves held diverse views on eugenics, and their political commitments ran the entire gamut from left to right (Rapp, 1999: 36). While eugenics appears to have been supported by many, if not most, scientists of the era, some scientists were harshly critical of the scientific methods and ideology of eugenics; i.e. its racism and class bias (Buchanan *et al.*, 2000: 35).

As Buchanan *et al.* conclude from their survey of the history of eugenics, if there was a core belief common to all eugenicists, it can be expressed in only the most general terms: concern for human betterment through selection (2000: 42). The level of generality of this characteristic of eugenics casts doubt on the validity of typifying eugenics as many proponents of the new genetics have done, and hence on their ability to draw a firm line between the 'new' genetics and the 'old' eugenics. It leads us to consider how appeals to differences based upon the 'new'/'old' dichotomy may serve a political and rhetorical purpose. In order to talk about 'essential' differences one needs to posit the 'new' genetics and the 'old' eugenics as unitary entities, with mutually exclusive goals, strategies, practices, and effects, thus denying the diversity of viewpoints and practices within each, as well as continuities in perspective, objectives, methods, and outcomes. The decision to focus on differences rather than similarities or continuities is a value judgement: one can select any set of criteria as evidence of difference, and overlook other criteria that show similarity or continuity. Differences are most apparent at the level of terminology. Writers often point to differences in language, which seem obvious: for example, the eugenic terms 'feeblemindedness', 'racial hygiene' and 'improvement of the stock' seem far removed from the 'new' genetic notions of 'right to know' and 'freedom of choice'. However, as others have argued, if one focuses on broad legitimizing rationales, use of particular strategies and practices, and effects or potential effects, one can identify a number of similarities and continuities between the 'new' genetics and the 'old' eugenics.

Similarities and continuities between the 'new' genetics and the 'old' eugenics: the public health connection

For a start, the legitimizing rationales employed by eugenicists seem not too dissimilar to those used by contemporary public health geneticists. Like them, eugenicists often portrayed their movement as a campaign for public health. There was in fact a great deal of overlap in programmes and personalities between the eugenics and public health movements, and much sharing of jargon. Thus, each resorted to the isolation and sterilization of the individuals who were thought to pose a threat to 'the public' (Buchanan *et al.*, 2000: 52). Those who were thought to harbour 'defective germ plasm' (what would now be called 'bad genes') were likened to carriers of infectious diseases. As Buchanan *et al.* explain:

While persons infected with cholera were a menace to those
with whom they came into contact, individuals with defective
germ plasm were an even greater threat to society: They transmitted harm to an unlimited number of persons across many
generations. The only difference between the 'horizontally
transmitted' infectious diseases and 'vertically transmitted'
genetic diseases, according to this view, was that the potential
harm caused by the latter was even greater.

(Buchanan *et al.*, 2000: 12)

The practice of quarantine, developed in nineteenth century public
health and involving the isolation of affected subgroups, would
seem to find its parallel in modern practices of genetic screening. In
Markel's (1992) view, the recent move to implement genetic
screening programmes on a wide scale reflects a 'quarantine
mentality', or the desire of society to separate itself from feared or
'undesirable' groups of people that was also evident in earlier,
eugenics practices. However, 'the new mark of "uncleanliness" is
not the telltale spots of the leper or the buboes of the plague that
once sounded the call for quarantine', but rather 'the positive result
of a genetic screening test, whether one actually has the disease or is
only a carrier' (Markel, 1992: 214). Observed similarities in the
practices and/or effects of the old eugenics and the new genetics
have prompted some writers to conclude that there is no essential
difference between the old eugenics and the new genetics.
Consequently, the latter has been dubbed 'the new eugenics' (e.g.
Allen, 1996, 1999; Duster, 1990; King, 1995; Rifkin, 1998: 127–8).

Jeremy Rifkin, for instance, refers to the new genetics as the 'new
eugenics', arguing that 'genetic engineering tools are, by definition,
eugenics instruments'. Any attempt to improve human beings,
animals or plants involves eugenic decisions, he says, since whenever
genetic change is made, the scientist, corporation or state is implicitly, if not explicitly, making decisions about the positive or negative
value of genes. However, this new 'user friendly' eugenics is being
presented as a social and economic boom. Instead of rhetoric about
racial purity, the new eugenics employs pragmatic terms such as
increased economic efficiency, better performance standards, and
improvement in the quality of life. While the old eugenics is seen as
imbued with political ideology and motivated by hate and fear, the
new eugenics is driven by market forces and consumer desire
(Rifkin, 1998: 128; see also King, 1995). Troy Duster (1990)

contends that the new genetic technologies have laid the foundation for the reincarnation of eugenics via 'the back door'. By this, Duster means that eugenic ends will be achieved not through coercive state policies based on claims of racial superiority or purity, but rather via a more indirect and subtle route; namely, the routine use of genetic screens, treatments, and therapies. In other words, eugenics is the unintended result of individual choices, and will happen under the guise of technical neutrality and medical benefit. In Duster's view, the availability of new genetic technologies will create pressures to use them, and the mere existence of the idea of a screen will infiltrate people's consciousness and communicate that the screened-for characteristic is undesirable. Articles such as 'The state of eugenics' (King, 1995), 'Eugenics revisited' (Horgan, 1993), and 'Science misapplied: the eugenics age revisited' (Allen, 1996) also voice the belief that the new genetic screening technologies are, in essence, eugenic. The only difference now, these writers suggest, is that the 'new eugenics' will be more subtle and will work via the market rather than via the state, and will be undertaken in the name of health.

The disability rights movement has tended to equate new genetics with Nazi-style eugenics. However, Tom Shakespeare (1998), a UK-based disability rights activist, has presented a more complex and nuanced analysis of the new genetic technologies. It is his view that in Britain at least, while eugenic views are held by some practitioners, particularly obstetricians, current genetics practice cannot be regarded as being strongly eugenic in the sense of being 'population-level improvement by control of reproduction via state intervention' (1998: 669). However, the pressures on women to undertake genetic testing, which is presented as a routine procedure, and to act on the results casts doubt on the capacity for informed consent and individual choice. Having had a test, women are subject to further pressures if it indicates the presence of a foetal abnormality, including pressure to take the decision to abort, which is the only possible 'action' other than doing nothing. Moreover, for some women choice is constrained by socioeconomic circumstances that limit the ability to care for the disabled child (1998: 675–7). This evidence leads Shakespeare to conclude that 'current British genetic practices are weakly, but not strongly, eugenic'. However, while there is strong rhetorical commitment to individual choice, the extension of screening to the whole population, combined with the tendency to frame screening policies in terms of cost-benefit analyses, may shift the balance towards 'strong eugenics' (1998: 669). (See Chapter 7.)

In the view of some writers, market forces are moving us inexorably towards a 'techno-eugenic' future, which will be legitimized in terms of the preventive benefits for the population as a whole. Thus, while the purported focus of 'new' genetics is on the benefits for the individual (e.g. 'somatic therapies'), attention is increasingly focused on the population gene pool (e.g. 'germ line therapies'). Rifkin (1998), for example, has noted that arguments are being advanced to develop germ line therapies, in terms of both the supposed preventive benefits for future populations and the expected cost savings in the longer term. In his view, prenatal testing has laid much of the philosophical groundwork for the acceptance of germ line therapy and 'a new commercial eugenics era' (1998: 131–3). Hayes (2000) has pointed to recent developments that suggest that the stage has been set for germ line manipulations which 'go beyond disease prevention and modify the genetic endowment of children otherwise expected to be healthy'. By the late 1990s, he says, proponents of germ line manipulations – what he calls the 'techno-eugenic lobby', comprising powerful biotech firms – have sought to persuade the public that attempts to restrict the use of human genetic technologies would represent an infringement of individual rights. For example, they have set up a series of programmes and institutes whose function it is to encourage public acceptance of the techno-eugenic technologies, including a major conference (which 'removed the taboo from advocacy of germline engineering') held at UCLA in 1998 and attended by 1,000 people (Hayes, 2000: 33–4).

There is indeed evidence to support the contention that the idea of germ line intervention is becoming more acceptable, and is being argued for on the grounds of future health benefits. For example, a recent edited collection, *Engineering the Human Germline: An Exploration of the Science and Ethics of Altering the Genes We Pass to Our Children*, contains contributions in which authors argue the case for 'germ line engineering' (Stock and Campbell, 2000). In one of the published panel discussions, James Watson, the co-discoverer of the structure of the DNA and former director of the National Centre for Human Genome Research of the National Institutes of Health, notes:

It seems obvious that germline therapy will be much more successful than somatic. If we wait for the success of somatic therapy, we'll wait until the sun burns out. We might as well do what we finally can to take the threat of Alzheimer's away from a family or breast cancer away from a family. The biggest ethical problem we have is not using our knowledge, ... people not having the guts to go ahead and try and help someone. We are always going to have to take some chances. It seems to me the question we're going to have to face is, what is going to be the least unpleasant? Using abortion to get rid of nasty genes from families? Or developing germline procedures with which, using Mario Capecchi's [a Professor of Human Genetics] techniques, you can go in and get rid of a bad gene.

(Part 2, The Road Ahead: A Panel Discussion, in Stock and Campbell, 2000: 79).

The expression of sentiments such as these are interpreted by critics of the new genetic technologies as evidence that we are already on the 'slippery slope' to eugenics (e.g. Rifkin, 1998: 133). As some writers argue, the line between germ line gene therapy (the attempt to restore health, or bring the patient back to 'normal') and enhancement genetic engineering (where one tries to improve 'normal') has become increasingly blurred. Indeed, at least one author in the above collection argues that they can see no reason for not allowing enhancement therapy, in view of pressing problems of environmental pollution, population explosion, the shortage of fossible fuels, and 'the serious lack of leadership' (Koshland, 2000: 29). He asks: 'Should we turn our back on new methodologies that might bring us smarter people and better leaders who are more responsible in their lives?' (Koshland, 2000: 29). One writer argues that justification for the use of germ line gene therapy is more likely to be made in terms of genetic enhancement, rather than in terms of alleviating disease, which involves mutations in single genes. Furthermore, it is suggested that pressure to use the therapies will come not from governments but from parents who wish to improve the chances for their biological children (Capecchi, 2000: 32). As the technologies of reproductive biology and genetics converge (i.e. 'reprogenetics'), 'prospective parents will gain the power to select which of their genes to pass down to their children and whether to add in other genes to protect their children from diseases, both inherited and infectious' (Silver, 2000: 67).

The context of the new genetics

One broad conclusion that can be drawn from the above work is that, increasingly, decisions about the development and applications of genetics are subject to the rationality of the market. That is, considerations of profitability, efficiency, 'consumer choice', and effective management have become increasingly evident in the justification for the development and use of genetic technologies. Indeed, some writers have observed strong parallels between the economic and social context giving rise to the new genetics and that which gave rise to the 'old' eugenics: that is, rising unemployment, falling average weekly incomes, and debates over health care (Allen, 1996: 29). As Allen notes, in Germany and the US between 1890 and 1930 eugenic ideas arose as a manifestation of what has been termed 'the search for order', involving attempts to bring a *laissez-faire* economy, and its related political and social practices, under control. The progressive ideology of the day called for the rational planning and scientific management of every phase of society, and used trained experts to set economic and social regulatory practices. It preached the doctrine of efficiency, applied cost-benefit analyses, and emphasized preventive rather than remedial measures, as in preventive medicine (1996: 27).

In Allen's view, the parallels between the contemporary economic and social situation in the US and that of Germany in the Weimar and Nazi periods are especially evident in debates over health care:

> Then as now, the discussions centred on decisions about who should receive what kind of care and for how long. Indeed in Germany medicine was considered a national resource to be used only for those individuals who showed the greatest prospects of recovery and future productivity. In the 'cutback' atmosphere that dominates our discussions of other social policies, the mood seems similarly exclusionary and bitter. For example, legislation that proposes to limit welfare recipients to five years over the lifetime, the suggestion that welfare mothers with more than two children be given Norplant (an antifertility drug), the idea of 'three strikes and you're out' (three convictions means a life sentence), and increasing calls for the death penalty – all run strikingly parallel to the mood of late Weimar and Nazi Germany that called for reduction of rations for, and later elimination of, the aged, those with terminal diseases,

repeat offenders, and the mentally impaired. Such measures were justified in Germany by the policy of efficiency and scarcity of resources. Our current focus on 'tough love' may be just a euphemism for what may somewhere down the road become 'lives not worth living'.

(1996: 29–30)

More recently, Allen (1999) has explored the context for the rise of genetic theories of human behaviour, and more specifically violence, again drawing parallels with the earlier eugenic period. In his view, current economic problems such as high unemployment, wage and benefit cuts, and increased urban violence, together with the publicity about the medical benefits flowing from advances in molecular genetics, particularly those associated with the HGP, help shape the context in which genetic determinist ideas have gained credence. Unlike the eugenics period, however, when attempts were made to legislate and control breeding patterns, advocates now focus on medical and technical means, including drug treatments and, if the technology becomes available, gene therapy. Although the techniques might vary somewhat – 'today's genetic determinists base their arguments more on statistical analyses of variance between identical twins or siblings in adoption studies, while the older eugenicists based their analyses largely on family pedigrees' – the two 'movements' share a similar function. That is, in both cases claims were made about the ability to treat complex and otherwise traditionally intractable social problems as amenable to solution through new 'scientific methods'. Under the mask of technical neutrality, the new genetics seems to offer simple solutions to complex problems, thereby diverting attention from the need to change the economic and social *status quo*. The victim in these circumstances is seen as the cause of his or her problems, and the simplest way to deal with those problems is to 'fix' them by scientific means. Genetic determinist arguments provide the rationale for an economically more 'efficient' (i.e. less expensive) way of dealing with so-called defective individuals (Allen, 1999: 17–18).

As Miringoff (1991) argues, a distinctive world view and new policies are evolving with the new genetic technologies that parallel the rolling back of the welfare state and increasing attacks on marginalized groups and minority rights. This world view challenges socially oriented perspectives, and reflects the notion that the public good is best served not by social intervention but by genetic or biological intervention. Miringoff uses the term Genetic Welfare to serve as a contrast to Social Welfare. As she explains:

> Social welfare, historically, has sought to improve human life by alterations in the social environment, through organizational and institutional change. In the Social Welfare perspective, problems are seen as embedded in society; solutions are typically located in the social structure. In Genetic Welfare, by contrast, change is sought at the genetic level; its purpose to improve the human species. In this definition, Genetic Welfare reflects a relative emphasis. It is not so much the total dominance of genetic considerations that is at issue, but their rising significance. ... In an array of issues involving birth, death, disease, disability, and the quality of life, we may now have to choose between genetic and social interventions. This choice is tilting toward the genetic, reflecting a shift in our vision of our abilities.
>
> (Miringoff, 1991: 6)

As evidence of this shift in world view, Miringoff observes that the focus in social welfare institutions on the support, training, and rehabilitation of the ill and disabled appears to be declining in favour of the new imperative of genetic prevention and genetic intervention. The burden of the genetically ill is viewed as redundant where the possibility exists of pursuing other paths. This has led to a reconsideration of our social responsibilities and changing perception of rights and duties. As Miringoff explains: 'Individuals are seen as having a *right* to genetic health; parents have a *duty* to ensure this outcome' (1991: 13; emphases in original). The technological ability to accomplish these outcomes presents a new imperative to ensure our genetic wellbeing. Although the means of introduction of the new genetics differs from that of early twentieth century eugenics, it does not necessarily differ in terms of substance. The main difference is that, unlike the eugenics movement, the genetic world view is 'neither religious nor messianic in tone' (1991: 29). For critics of the new genetic technologies, the main problem is not fervour but indifference. New genetic and reproductive technologies have become a routine, and hence an unexceptional, part of everyday technical and administrative decisions, and are posed not as efforts to change the world or civilization, as was the case with eugenics, but as means to improve our health and wellbeing (1991: 29–30). The legitimacy medicine offers to genetic and reproductive technologies has been crucial to the emergence of Genetic Welfare. Medicine contributes to public acceptance of the new genetic technologies, and may serve as a conduit for channelling genetic ideas beyond medicine into other arenas. Genetic screening creates new modes of labelling and stigma, and reinforces the search for perfection and hence intolerance of difference (e.g. people with disabilities) (1991: 30–4, 47–62).

The impact of the genetic world view on the field of public health: international, regional, and local manifestations

The argument that we have entered a period in which the genetic world view is becoming more prominent would seem to be borne out by recent developments in the field of public health. In the 1990s diverse public health authorities, at both the national and international level, made concerted efforts to improve the 'genetic literacy' of health providers and the general population, and to apply genetic approaches for the prevention and management of a rapidly expanding range of diseases. This period, dominated by what some scholars describe as 'neo-liberal' forms of rule, has been one of rapid change that has seen a withdrawal of many nation states from their commitment to welfare provision, and an increased liberalization of markets, involving the rapid transnational flow of people, trade, and information. While nation states have not completely abrogated responsibility for social provision and social intervention, there is evidence of increased focus on genetic or biological explanations of many health and social problems previously seen as amenable to social structural solutions. In recent years there have been incessant calls for health workers to become *au fait* with the role of genetics in health and disease, and for relevant experts and organizations to collaborate locally, regionally, and internationally to promote health through genetic approaches and to improve genetic health education. Conferences involving public health practitioners and other specialists have aimed to enhance awareness about the scope and processes for integrating genetic knowledge into public health programmes and to strengthen partnerships in pursuit of disease prevention (see, for example, Gettig *et al.*, 1999; Khoury *et al.*, 1998; Khoury *et al.*, 2000). In the public health and medical literature, practitioners have been advised about the importance of understanding the fundamentals of genetic epidemiology and of the ability to accurately assess the genetic risk of individuals and families, and about the necessity of gaining knowledge of disease prevention strategies and programmes (see, for example, Fineman, 1999; Hayflick and Eiff, 1998: 19). At the same time, efforts have been made to increase general public awareness of genetic health and disease through such means as consensus conferences, citizens' juries, genetic support groups, and advertising at strategic locations (e.g. the Gene Shop at Manchester Airport, UK) (Glasner and Dunkerley, 1999; Kinmonth et al., 1998: 769). (See Chapter 7.)

With the increasing liberalization of markets and the relative weakening of nation states and a lessening of their commitment to the provision of health and welfare services, many important initiatives in genetic disease prevention are occurring at the supranational level. New communication technologies, particularly the Internet, have assisted communications across national borders and given rise to new 'virtual communities'. There has been an exponential growth of genetic resources on the Web, oriented to both health care providers and lay publics; for example, genetic discussion forums and information on specific diseases and genetic support groups (see, for example, Gettig et al., 1999: 120; Kinmonth et al., 1998: 768; Rose and Lucassen, 1999: 347–8). These websites often serve a broad networking and educative purpose, in that they assist in the formation of new international links and the dissemination of genetic knowledge in general, in addition to offering a resource on specific genetic conditions and resources for particular interested groups. An example of using the web in such a way is the Human Genome Epidemiology Network (HuGE Net), which involves a 'collaboration of individuals from diverse backgrounds who are committed to the development and dissemination of population-based human genome epidemiological information' (Khoury, 1998). HuGE Net has developed an 'updated and accessible knowledge base' on the Web, and seeks to promote the use of this knowledge by health care providers, researchers, industry and the public for disease prevention and health promotion (Khoury, 1998: 100). The dissemination of genetic ideas at the international level has been advanced substantially by the World Health Organization (WHO), through its Human Genetics Programme (HGN). In recent years, WHO has taken the initiative in developing genetic approaches for the prevention and control of common hereditary diseases and genetic risk, and in forging networks of international collaborating programmes, centres and experts (Boulyjenkov, 1998). With the financial support and cooperation of various non-government and international organizations (e.g. the Thalassaemia International Federation, the International Cystic Fibrosis (Mucoviscidosis) Association, the International Clearing House for Birth Defects Monitoring Systems), as well as the pharmaceutical industry, the WHO has embarked on an ambitious programme of education and training.

WHO is providing international expertise and technical advice to countries for a number of activities, and organizes meetings to discuss research developments and experiences of ongoing national programmes. It provides educational materials and guidelines on the principles of the formation of national programmes for the control of genetic diseases, and supports and organizes training courses on the principles and organization of community control programmes and methods of diagnostic procedures (Boulyjenkov, 1998: 58). Haemoglobin disorders (thalassaemia and sickle cell disorder (SCD)), in particular, have been identified as the focus of control programmes, and as 'a convenient model for working out an approach to control chronic childhood diseases in developing countries' (1998: 57). As Boulyjenkov points out, approximately 4.5 per cent of the world's population carries the haemoglobinopathy gene and, each year, about 300,000 infants are born with a major haemoglobin disorder. A majority (70 per cent) of cases of SCD occurs in sub-Saharan Africa, where up to 2 per cent of children are born with the disorder. With increasing global migration, it is argued, the disorders have been introduced into many areas where they were not originally endemic; for example, the USA and north-west Europe (1998: 57). The effort to stem the spread of genetic (i.e. 'vertically transmitted') diseases from the Third World to the First World through control programmes mirrors the 'traditional' public health effort to control the spread of infectious ('horizontally transmitted') diseases from the working classes to the upper classes through quarantine. Recommendations have been established for each WHO Region (Africa, the Americas, the Eastern Mediterranean, Europe, South-East Asia, the Western Pacific). With these programmes having been deemed 'successful', new thalassaemia and SCD programmes are being developed in a number of countries, including Brazil, China, Greece, India, Italy,

Myanmar, Pakistan, Thailand, Tunisia, Turkey, the UK, Cuba, Jamaica, and Nigeria. Drawing on this experience, the WHO is now turning its attention to other prevalent genetic diseases such as cystic fibrosis, haemophilia, neurofibromatosis and haemochromatosis (1998: 57–8).

In light of an expected substantial increase in demand for genetic information and advice, geneticists and public health practitioners have called for the reorganization of existing genetic services and the integration of new genetic knowledge into routine practice. Primary health care providers (e.g. doctors, nurses, audiologists) are seen to play a key role, as 'front line' workers, in the effort to detect the genetically susceptible and 'carriers' of genetic defects, and to facilitate 'clients' use of genetic services. Given their traditional focus on the family unit, their long-term involvement with individuals, and their use of counselling techniques in practice, they are seen as particularly well placed to apply genetic information (Harris *et al.*, 1999). The *British Medical Journal* recently carried a number of articles exploring the impacts of the new genetics on clinical services and suggesting how genetic information may be integrated into practice in the 'post-genome' era (e.g. Bell, 1998; Gill and Richards, 1998; Kinmonth *et al.*, 1998). Among other things, there have been demands for collaboration between geneticists, public health specialists, and primary care teams (Gill and Richards, 1998: 570). Writers frequently lament the inadequacy of practitioner training in genetics, with predictions that, without urgent action, 'crisis' is inevitable:

> Genetics holds a unique position in medicine. Genetic factors contribute to nearly every common disease, yet most physicians, nurses and other health care providers have had only limited, if any training in genetics. This lack of training has already had harmful consequences, which have been limited in scale. As genetic testing pervades routine health care, the repercussions of this disparity between training provided and knowledge required will worsen. Our challenge is to stimulate improved training at all levels before a crisis is upon us.
>
> (Hayflick and Eiff, 1998: 18)

As these and other writers argue, genetic risk assessment should become a part of routine care, along with the provision of other services (Bell, 1998: 619; Harris *et al.*, 1999; Hayflick and Eiff,

1998: 19–20). In the UK, there is already evidence of increased interest in and demand for such services from patients and practitioners, especially where regional centres are developing new services and raising awareness and expectations. Such awareness is even greater in the US, where websites and private genetics services promote genetic issues and opportunities for testing (Kinmonth *et al.*, 1998: 768).

In Europe, concerns about the inability of genetic services to cope with existing and expanding workloads led the European Commission to establish the Concerted Action on Genetic Services in Europe (CAGSE), with the aim of assessing the current state of specialist genetics services. Drawing on data from a survey undertaken in 1996 in thirty-one countries in the European Union, former Soviet bloc and eastern Mediterranean region, CAGSE identified a number of problems in services. These included inadequate or inappropriate teaching and training of genetics staff, lack of trained counsellors, and regional inequalities in the provision of services. CAGSE recommended the development of a European charter for national medical genetics societies, with a broad interdisciplinary membership responsible for, among other things, strategic planning for developing services, networking between genetics centres both nationally and internationally, and advising on the clinical and public health applications of genetic discoveries. In addition, it recommended the integration of regional genetics centres, enhanced cooperation between the various clinical, laboratory, and psycho-social aspects of the services, and the expeditious development of training programmes for genetic workers, 'including provision of accurate empathic genetic counseling in connection with genetic tests' (Harris *et al.*, 1999: 50).

Initiatives such as these highlight the increasing significance attached to genetic health at both the national and international level, and the new forms of social organization and activity that are emerging in response to the effort to manage genetic risk. International, regional, and local networks involving interdisciplinary and inter-organizational collaborations are beginning to reshape the field of public health, and to give rise to new imperatives surrounding health, risk, and preventive action. This increasing attention to improving 'genetic literacy' and to providing services for detecting and counselling the genetically 'at risk' is redefining the norms of health and is bound to affect people's subjective experience of their own sense of wellbeing, vulnerability, and control. As more and more diseases are identified as having a genetic component, a growing number of individuals will be identified, or will come to identify themselves, as being genetically 'at risk' or as having 'carrier' status. That is, people's social identities and social actions will be increasingly tied to knowledge about their genetic makeup.

New citizenship rights and duties implied by genetic risk management

The shifts in world view discussed above are reflected in the imperatives of citizenship and involve new individual rights and duties in relation to genetic health and risk. The unstated assumption underlying the effort to promote people's genetic literacy is that not only do people have a right to genetic information, but they also have a *duty* to minimize or manage their own contribution to genetic disease. In line with new public health thinking and the imperatives of active citizenship more generally, citizens are *expected* to participate in the advancement of their own health and wellbeing (Petersen and Lupton, 1996: 146–73). They should be aware of the role of genetics in health and disease in general and in their own health in particular, know what services are available to assist them, and take appropriate preventive action. These norms of citizenship are reflected in the rhetoric of the 'right to know' and 'informed choice'. The guiding premise is that people can only act autonomously if their decision-making is 'informed'; that is, if they 'know' what their own genetic risk is and what their options are. This strong emphasis on the right to knowledge and 'freedom of choice' is strongly evident in contemporary public health literature, and is seen as a characteristic that clearly distinguishes the new genetics from the earlier eugenics programmes. The eugenic policies pursued by many states in the past – a programmatic effort to alter the heredity substance at the level of populations – are considered anathema to the prevailing orthodoxy of neo-liberalism. In societies characterized by 'governance through freedom' (N. Rose, 1999), there is little tolerance for the degree of state intervention that is generally associated with the era of eugenics.

The expectation is that the individual will inform themselves about their genetic risk, and take whatever steps are deemed necessary to reduce the risk to themselves and to others, especially if they are found to be a 'carrier' and a prospective parent. Clearly, obligations associated with genetic risk management always have an inter-generational dimension (see below). Arguments for wider public access to genetic knowledge, steeped as they are in the language of rights and freedoms – 'right to know' and 'freedom of choice' – always carry the expectation that, once 'informed', the individual will act 'responsibly' through exercising 'choice'. Indeed, they are *compelled* to choose. Moreover, 'choice' is not unconstrained: it is constrained by the available preventive or treatment options (often very limited), and the broader social context, including socioeconomic conditions, ethnicity, religion, the individual's family relations, and personal and cultural views on parenthood.

The assumption of the 'right to know' and 'informed choice' is clearly apparent, for example, in a recent discussion of 'ethical and philosophical issues raised by developments in genetic screening techniques' in Europe (Chadwick and Levitt, 1996). A Danish Council of Ethics report noted that 'there is an obligation to help the weak which will be best exemplified when screening results in the curing of the disease' and that, 'in genetics, the duty of help has a special intention – to offer information that will facilitate autonomy'. This argument is based on the paternalistic premise that experts know what is best for individuals and that some hypothetical end ('cure') justifies the means (screening). It does not address the question of exactly how genetic information can 'facilitate autonomy' and, indeed, what is meant by 'autonomy' and what personal and interpersonal rights and responsibilities this implies, nor does it consider whether people have a right not to know (Chadwick *et al.*, 1997). The assumed relation between genetic information and 'autonomy' has been the subject of extensive critique in recent years, particularly on the grounds of the failure to acknowledge the effect of the social context on both the interpretation and exercise of 'autonomy' (see, for example, Huibers and van 't Spijker, 1998; White, 1999). However, the assumption that 'knowledge is a good thing', and 'the more knowledge the better', remains largely undisputed in the new genetics, and underpins the 'non-directive' approach of genetic counselling. (See Chapter 5.) In the expert literature, there has been little acknowledgement of the fact that genetic information is complex and difficult to interpret, that experts may disagree about the significance of test results, and that the results of diagnostic tests can be more confusing than helpful (Feldman, 1996). Difficulties in interpreting genetic information are compounded by rapid changes in the practice of genetic screening, as it assimilates the findings of the HGP and other 'gene-mapping' initiatives. In prenatal genetic counselling, decisions are often based on partial information – perhaps nothing more than a probability resulting from a research-stage test – under severe time constraints (Malinowski, 1994). Such complexities and difficulties tend to be overlooked or downplayed in many discussions about the new genetics and its public health implications, which simply take it as given that where genetic information is seen to exist, citizens need it and experts can and should provide it. We explore in more detail in the final chapter how these citizenship imperatives impact upon the lives of those who have thus far been affected most directly by new genetic technologies, and how these groups have responded.

'The family' as a factor of risk and site for preventive intervention

One important insight provided by the new genetics is the significance of the family as a 'factor of risk' and site for preventive intervention. It has long been observed that some diseases seem to 'run in families'. However, as many geneticists themselves acknowledge, it is difficult to be certain whether this is because members of the same family tend to share the same environment or whether there is a genetic cause of the disease (see, for example, Russo and Cove, 1995: 105). Molecular technologies are being applied in studies of families to identify disease and 'susceptibility' genes. These studies, which are mostly based on 'high-risk' families where many individuals are affected, have led to the identification of, most notably, the breast cancer genes (Khoury, 1996: 1717). The importance of knowing the 'family history' or 'pedigree' for preventive action is emphasized in the recent public health and primary health care literature, and in advice offered to prospective parents or to those concerned about their carrier status or genetic disease risk. As an article appearing in the *British Medical Journal* notes: 'Obtaining good family history data is an essential start in the assessment and management of genetic disorders' (Kinmonth *et al.*, 1998: 769).

Given their ascribed position as leaders of 'the primary health care team', general practitioners are seen to play a crucial role in eliciting a family history and assisting in the promotion of 'family-focused' preventive action. Recent texts on genetics and primary care advise practitioners about the importance of the pedigree as a diagnostic tool, and how it can be developed from the existing family history that doctors elicit in the course of consultations. As one writer (a GP) explains, the pedigree can:

- alert a family to the possibility that there are genetic factors running through the family;
- be used to establish the type of inheritance;
- help to estimate the risk to individuals that they may be a gene carrier or the likelihood that they will develop a given disease.

(P. Rose, 1999: 57)

Eliciting a family tree, it is argued, will allow practitioners to differentiate 'low-risk' and 'high-risk' patients, and either to offer reassurance to the former or to refer the latter to medical geneticists for further advice. However, as practitioners themselves recognize, there are few proven interventions to offer patients deemed to be at high risk (P. Rose, 1999: 61). For women who are found to have inherited the gene mutation linked to breast cancer, for example, the only available means of primary prevention thus far has been prophylactic mastectomy, which may not provide full protection against the development of breast cancer (Khoury, 1996: 1718). As the above text notes, the task of eliciting the family tree need not involve practitioners in face-to-face communication with the patient, since it may be delegated to other members of the primary health team. (It points out that it is common practice in clinical genetics departments to delegate the task to nurses.) Furthermore, patients can be contacted before their appointment and asked to fill in a detailed 'family history questionnaire', which will enable the doctor to construct the pedigree before the consultation, or they can be 'instructed beforehand to find out all the information they can about their family history' (P. Rose, 1999: 67). It is anticipated that, in the future, all family histories will be undertaken with the aid of computers. Indeed, as Rose points out, there are already computer programs that will draw up a pedigree and evaluate risks, and programs are being developed that will integrate family history taking into the general practice software that runs on the GP's desktop computer (P. Rose, 1999: 67).

More and more, people are being advised about the importance of knowing their family's history and of initiating their own research into the illnesses afflicting relatives, with a view to uncovering possible genetic-linked disease. In the health promotion and self-help literature one can find advice on how to draw a family tree, and how to find out if there are any hereditary conditions in the family. The Internet has also become a source of advice in this respect (see, for example, www.genetics.com.au; www.progeny2000. com). Knowing one's pedigree is presented as having future preventive benefits, for both oneself and one's family. As the book, *Genetic Nutrition* explains:

> Constructing a health family tree is an act of discovery, a kind of genetic sleuthing that can improve your future health, and the health of your family as well. While it cannot erase concerns about illnesses that are not primarily genetic, it can produce significant red flags pointing to inherited conditions. If such warnings turn up in your family tree, you and your relatives can seek medical advice early, and perhaps prevent or delay the onset of disease. Such care may include everything from lifestyle changes like weight loss, regular exercise, and alterations in how much you eat and the foods you choose, to drug therapy to reduce cholesterol or blood pressure. The 'tree' may not only identify the diseases that have turned up in your family's past, but also indicate how they have been transmitted through the generations, and identify those family members who may be at risk of getting them now or in the future.
>
> (Simopolous *et al.*, 1993: 33)

The authors provide a detailed account of 'what to look for' (including illness or conditions that relatives have (or have had)), 'how to gather information' (using a health questionnaire), and how to organize the data in a form that is useful to a physician or genetic counsellor. It also notes that it is important 'to be a careful detective if you are a member of an ethnic group which is susceptible to a specific genetic disease'. Advice is given on the particular conditions that one should investigate if one is a member of any of the groups mentioned; namely, Jewish, African-American, Japanese, and Irish (Simopolous *et al.*, 1993: 34–51).

The use of the family tree or pedigree has a long history, having been part of the technology of the eugenic movement in the early twentieth century (Kevles, 1995: 45–6). Such family trees were often based on highly subjective and impressionistic data collected from family members, and informed by a naïve understanding of genetics and inheritance (Allen, 1996: 24). Given that constructing the family history involves questions that are usually about events in the past, and necessitates reliance on old records, recollections of family members, and patients' own evaluations, the value of the data as a diagnostic tool is in doubt. Practitioners themselves sometimes admit the problem of drawing conclusions from potentially 'inaccurate' information arising from, for example, reliance on details from death certificates, patients' confusion of diagnoses, or lack of knowledge of important diagnoses. Furthermore, a family history is open to different interpretations, depending on the reasons why it has been taken in the first place. If one is concerned about the possibility of a single gene disorder running through a family, the interpretation of the family tree will focus on that disease alone. On the other hand, if no particular diagnosis is suspected, then the family will be scrutinized for a diagnosis or a group of diagnoses running through the tree which could potentially be explained by one genetic abnormality (see, for example, P. Rose, 1999: 68–9).

Questions can also be raised about how information may be used. There is no suggestion at present that data derived from family trees will be used in an intentional way for neo-eugenic purposes. However, given that health planners see data on 'family risk' as playing an increasingly important role in the management of genetic disease within populations – as 'facilitat[ing] rational planning and provision of genetic services' (Genetic Services of Western Australia, 1995) – there exists the potential for this data to at least provide the basis for new insidious forms of 'family'-focused technologies of surveillance and control. The comments and suggestions outlined in a recent report by the Nuffield Council on Bioethics are significant in this regard (Gillon, 1994). As the Council indicated, the individual who has been screened and is found to have a genetic disorder has a responsibility to other family members who may be carriers, knowledge of which might alter family members' approach to reproduction (for example, in the case of cystic fibrosis, thallasaemia or Tay-Sachs disease), or who may themselves be at risk of a severe genetic disorder whose manifestations may be fatal and preventable (e.g breast cancer) or fatal and unpreventable (e.g. Huntington's disease). The Council suggests that where individuals are reluctant to pass on such information to other family members they may need to be 'persuaded' by health professionals to do so. And, where such 'persuasion' is unsuccessful, and the information is seen to 'have serious implications for relatives', they may even need to be denied rights to confidentiality.

Responsibility to one's family, it is clear, has a strong intergenerational dimension, encompassing one's distant and *potential* family members. Responsible family planning requires prospective parents to exercise appropriate forethought and carefully consider the risks and responsibilities that follow from the decision to have a genetic test. A pamphlet which advises on testing for birth defects in pregnancy, published by the Health Department of Western Australia, informs prospective parents that 'before deciding to have tests it is important to consider how you might personally feel if testing shows your baby to have a hereditary condition'. It notes that 'if a condition is found, a doctor or genetic counsellor will explain the implications to assist you and your partner in making a well informed decision', adding that 'you are free to make whatever decision you feel is right for you' (Hereditary Disease Unit, 1995). Prenatal genetic testing and counselling is becoming an accepted part of family planning and is presented as a necessary basis for 'informed' decision-making (see Rapp, 1999; Rothenberg and Thomson, 1994). Although costs presently dictate that testing tends to be limited to older parents and families where there is deemed to be an increased risk of a specific genetic condition, as it becomes cheaper and technologies improve genetic testing is likely to become incorporated into routine prenatal care (Gupta and Bianchi, 1997).

There is some evidence from the US that many physicians now view prenatal genetic tests as risk-free blood tests and either pressure women to undergo them or surreptitiously test pregnant women's blood for carrier status (Andrews, 1996). The range of tests offered is growing continually, due in large measure to the concerted efforts of the HGP and other gene-mapping initiatives. Prenatal tests are now available not just for life-threatening disorders but for conditions that are treatable after birth, for conditions that do not manifest until later in life, such as breast cancer, and for other non-medical problems, such as homosexuality. Clearly, the implications of these developments for 'choice' in reproductive decision-making are profound. In the future, self-testing for genetic disease may become routine, in much the same way as self-testing to confirm pregnancy now is. In Britain a company has already offered cystic fibrosis screening by post and, in the US, companies have offered genetic tests for predisposition to a variety of cancers, despite uncertainties about the significance of such test results (King, 1995). We may soon reach a situation where individuals are seen as irresponsible for not undergoing genetic tests where these are available (Crossley, 1996).

King predicts that, in the future, 'we are going to be told that if we know that certain genes cause disease and we can test for them, then we are being irresponsible leaving things to chance; and that we are being irresponsible and cruel if we even consider bringing a disabled child into the world' (1995: 25). As King explains:

> One way or the other, we are all going to be dragged into the regime of gene management, that will, in essence, be eugenic. It will all be in the name of individual health rather than for the overall fitness of the population, and the managers will be you and me and our doctors, and not the state. Genetic change will be managed by the invisible hand of individual choice, but the overall result will be the same, a co-ordinated attempt to 'improve' the genes of the next generation on the way.
>
> (King, 1995: 26)

The routinization of prenatal genetic testing and genetic counselling are likely to create the conditions for a 'eugenics of normalcy' (Keller, 1992: 299). That is, the collective actions of individuals exercising their 'right to normalcy' – to perfect health and to perfect offspring – may have eugenic consequences. It is noteworthy that, in discussions about the new genetics, the meaning of 'normal' is never defined and never constitutes the subject of debate. Indeed, the ambiguity residing in the very term 'normal' is the source of a potent power in that it suggests both that the normal is what is right and that there is something to be improved upon. As Keller argues, eugenics has become 'a vastly more realizable prospect' than it was in the early part of the twentieth century. However, the source of concern is not a Nazi-style racist policy, but rather 'our own complacency that there are some "right hands" in which to invest responsibility – above all, the responsibility for arbitrating normality' (1992: 299).

Conclusion

For a term that is so widely used, it is surprising how often writers either leave undefined, or only loosely define, 'the new genetics'. As has been argued in this chapter, in so far as 'the new genetics' is defined at all, it tends to be described in terms of its benefits in advancing individual autonomy and 'freedom of choice', and to be sharply distinguished from eugenics, which is associated with coercive control by the state. The 'new' in the term 'the new genetics' serves as a boundary marker, differentiating that which is seen as progressive, scientific, and liberating (i.e. personally 'empowering') from that which is deemed antiquated, pseudo-scientific, and repressive. However, as we have also shown, recent historical work, which exposes the diverse manifestations of eugenics, questions the validity of this dichotomy. According to this history, the commonality between the strands of eugenics can be expressed in only the most general terms: concern with human betterment. When eugenics is defined at this level of generality, there would seem to be continuities between 'the new genetics' and eugenics. Some writers, indeed, see them as having similar outcomes, leading them to dub the former 'the new eugenics'. However, an evident difference is that, whereas eugenics operated or operates largely via the authority of the state and makes reference to improvements in the health of the population, 'the new genetics' works predominantly through the mechanism of the market and uses the language of personal empowerment and 'consumer choice'.

Finally, this chapter has examined efforts to promote 'genetic literacy' at international, regional, and local levels. The growing liberalization of markets has undermined the autonomy of the nation state and, more and more, supranational organizations such as the WHO have taken a leading role in promoting the genetic world view at the global level, assisted by new communication technologies such as the Internet. Increasingly, people are expected, as part of their duties as citizens, to play their part in minimizing or managing their own contribution to genetic disease. An important element of genetic literacy, it was argued, is knowledge about one's family history, oriented to uncovering genetic-linked disease. Within the genetic world view, 'the family' is a primary factor of risk and site for preventive intervention. Meanwhile, the questions of whether or not genetics offers the most effective means of combating the diseases that are responsible for the majority of illnesses and disabilities suffered by people at the global level, and what the consequences of the genetic world view are for different groups, are largely overlooked. The notion that the individual is the source of, and is responsible for, managing disease, and that the socioeconomic system is essentially benign, sits comfortably with the premises of neo-liberalism described earlier. Arguably, the focus on genetic disease and intervention at the level of individuals and families diverts attention from social structural and global-level solutions that are urgently needed to reduce inequalities in health and wellbeing. The next chapter develops the argument further by placing genetic technologies in a broader context of technological change that is shaping our ways of seeing and living, and by examining the impact of genetic technologies on thinking and action in the field of public health in particular.

Chapter 3

Genes, technology, and public health

Robin Bunton

Making sense of the application of the new genetics to health and public health relates to our understanding of the role of new technology in the contemporary social world. Our discussion of the new genetics has highlighted the ways that emerging technologies of surveillance, epidemiology, diagnosis and treatment have implications for social relationships in relation to counselling practice and to the conceptions of citizenship. Here we present the new genetics as one of many technologies that are transforming modern societies. We argue that the new genetic knowledge and techniques are changing some of the fundamental concepts and practices of public health. Genetic technologies have consequences for the surveillance of the individual and populations. They have consequences for the environment and for the survival of potentially harmful 'agents' that threaten our health. In affecting all of these elements they bring into question some familiar features of public health. In this chapter we discuss the broad social implications of technology for industrial societies and how we can account for the place of new technologies. We then examine how gene technologies are introducing new ways of thinking and working within the field.

A significant feature of contemporary Western industrial societies is an increasing reliance on technology in manufacturing services, information processing, communication, education, health care and public administration. Technology was eagerly embraced by early supporters of modernity, such as Francis Bacon and René Descartes, who saw technology as central to the power of liberal democratic societies. The surplus wealth that technology made possible seemed to justify capitalist systems of production from the eighteenth century onwards. Since then, increasing dependence on technology has had a more mixed reception and is seen to be at the centre of a number of political problems and controversies. The social costs and ethical dilemmas of technology have been listed by Pippin (1994). Reliance on technology concentrates power in fewer hands and creates expert elites. The lack of public understanding of science and technology creates problems for accountability and decision-making. A narrowing of acceptable topics of public debate can often occur and collective decisions can be reduced to technical matters, resulting in a depoliticizing of many aspects of life. Labour forces can be deskilled through automation and other hierarchical forms of efficient administration. Increased administration of daily life, made possible by data storage in medicine, government, banking and insurance, can be manipulative and cumbersome. Finally, technology may dehumanize aspects of culture and the environment, involving, for example, the medicalization of birth, death and illness.

These concerns have introduced elements of public mistrust and even cynicism about science and technology. The more spectacular and promising the technology, the more disbelief becomes possible (Segal, 1994). The science and technology that once almost universally brought praise now brings mistrust and suspicion. In his aptly titled book *The Descent of Icarus* (1990), Ezrahi argues that the state's reliance on science and technology to justify intervention in most areas of public life has been undermined. Increased questioning of the authority of 'experts' would appear to be a feature of the last two decades. Some have argued that dispute and critique of science and scientific risk will ultimately reverse some anti-democratic tendencies of expert-led, technocratic social systems (Beck, 1992, 2000; Giddens, 1991). The hazards and risks imposed on the public will engender reflection, critique and ultimately more active participation and debate, resulting in democratization. Public concern about the arrival of new genetic technologies has also been widespread and might be seen as part of a broader tendency to question science and technology.

The relationship between technology and society is often complex, and criticism has been directed at those who have painted, and over-simplified, the 'technological determinist' picture, privileging the role of the scientists in discovering, disseminating and 'advancing' society (Ellul, 1964; Mumford, 1934). Recent work, however, has drawn attention to the ways in which society often determines technology, and the ways that technological systems and social systems are intertwined. Hill (1988), for example, made the case for exploring the 'culture defining power of technology', and considering technology as a type of 'cultural text'. Analysis of the processes of invention and innovation has stressed the complex and often subtle process of interactions between humans, techniques and technologies (Latour, 1992). Popular accounts of the development of genetic technologies (such as those discussed in Chapter 4) describe a technologically determined world in which social life is changed or 'advanced' by the introduction of new technologies. Medicine is about to be 'revolutionized', the human 'race' 'improved', and treatment and prevention changed through the actions of microbiological technologies. Such accounts ignore the social conditions that allow certain technological developments to occur at all. Much of the social history of science has pointed to the social shaping or social 'embeddedness' of technological process. The technologies of industrial production, for example, according to the analyses of Karl Marx (1967) or Max Weber (Whimster and Lash, 1987), were made possible by particular sets of social relationships and beliefs specific to seventeenth, eighteenth and nineteenth century Europe. The absence of these conditions in other parts of the world meant that capitalist production techniques and processes could not gain momentum. Such accounts turn technological deterministic accounts on their head and present instead a social determinist argument. More recent work in the sociology of science and technology has developed a more dynamic and interactive account of the relationship between technology and humans which may provide insights into the changing conceptions of health, health care and health management currently being brought about through work in genetics (Berg, 1997; Oudshoorn, 1994; Prout, 1996). Though there is great variety in the study of innovation and technological change, most contemporary approaches agree that the introduction of new technology involves social, economic, and political as well as technological processes, and that technology develops hand in hand with new sets of social relationships.

Most technological development is the outcome of the interaction of a number of key elements acting as a system. The history of the electricity industry illustrates this well. Thomas P. Hughes' analysis *Networks of Power*, as Law (2000) observes, charts the growth of the electricity industry, its production and organization of supply, as the outcome of the system building of entrepreneurs such as Thomas Edison. The system they built included not simply the technical elements necessary to make city-wide electricity, but also a series of equally necessary economic, legal and political components. While the technical development was indeed important (such as the creation of the incandescent light bulb), technical elements were inextricably mixed up with political deals, with local political agendas, and with:

> legal arrangements about the location of supply cables and generating stations, and economic calculations about how far (and at what voltages) it was profitable to transmit power before losses became unsustainable.
>
> (Law, 2000: 4)

Concern about 'over-technologizing' modern medicine has a long history (Cartwright, 1967). There has been some recent sociological concern about the 'sociotechnical networks' that exist in medical settings (Atkinson et al., 1997; Elston, 1997). Similarly, we can usefully see public health as a system of actors including people, governments, companies, entrepreneurs, technologies, environments and diseases. This system is constantly being reconfigured such that our conceptions of health, health policy and governance, prevention and cure are subject to change. The introduction of newer technologies, such as genetic technologies, is changing the configuration of this system. We have pointed to some of the ways that technological developments in genetics match and coincide with recent changes and developments in conceptions of health, preventive strategy and understandings of the responsibilities of the state and citizens. Certain ideas of genetic intervention appear to 'fit' or function well with techniques for monitoring and surveying populations seen to be 'at risk' and in need of prophylactic intervention. Genetic technology facilitates surveillance in ways that suit a particular health policy (as discussed in Chapter 6). The subject of contemporary health care regimes is expected to shoulder a larger responsibility for his or her own health than in previous generations and is expected to calculate and insure against such vulnerability personally, as the collective or public management of risk gives way to privatized risk management strategies. New forms of governance are facilitating the development of genetic technologies, as these technologies facilitate new forms of governance. We have drawn upon the work influenced by Michel Foucault, which draws attention to such changes in the construction of the contemporary subject.

Conceiving of technology as one aspect of a social-technical network draws attention to the often invisible work that maintains such networks (Leigh-Starr, 1991). Much of the power of technology lies in the fact that it can solidify or frame sets of social relationships in ways that are invisible or appear 'natural'. Technology can work in a similar way to ideology in this respect. It carries its own imperative, making its use seem somehow inevitable, unproblematical and rational. Technology is erroneously seen as value neutral. Rather it 'mediates' or frames everyday life and provides, as Heidegger (1949) observed, an 'orientation to being'.

Technology can purport a world view or a 'horizoning' of experience:

> This means that ... reliance [on technology] reaches a point where what ought to be understood as contingent, one option among others, open to political discussion, is instead falsely understood as a necessary (i.e. relevant options are not even noted as credible options: hence the 'false consciousness'); what serves particular interests is seen, without reflection, as of universal interest; what is a contingent, historical experience is regarded as natural; what ought to be part is experienced as the whole; and so on.
>
> (Pippin, 1994: 96–7)

Martin has recently drawn upon the sociology of science to examine the social shaping of gene therapy (Martin, 1999). Drawing on a range of recent approaches to the social study of technology, he notes that new technology development involves a variety of heterogeneous social, technical, economic and political processes. New knowledge is 'co-produced' at the same time as new technologies and new sociotechnical relations mutually shape one another. Martin focuses on the gene therapy, sociotechnical network developed by scientists, industrialists, politicians and other key actors over the last thirty years or so and identifies four major changes in the progression from idea to clinical reality. He plots a shift from eugenics in a series of stages towards a conception of gene therapy that is akin to contemporary concepts of drugs.

Firstly, the link to eugenics was broken when germ line therapy was ruled unethical, paving the way for the legitimate development of somatic therapy. The second change was the break with classical genetics that occurred when the first cancer trial was approved and classical gene therapy, for technical reasons, was abandoned as a serious option. This opened up the possibility of treating a wide range of acquired diseases through the development of cell implants. Following this, the next major transition was marked by the shift from gene therapy as an ex vivo surgical procedure to it becoming a form of *in vivo* drug delivery. Simultaneously, the technology was reconfigured to provide a temporary rather than a permanent cure.

(Martin, 1999: 534)

Each of the above transformations occurred as investigators struggled to build stable networks, and each subsequent stage involved the reconstitution of the concept of genetic disease. By reshaping the technology and the disease concept it was possible to obtain the support of all groups and the resources necessary to introduce gene therapy into the clinic.

Martin points to the key role played by actors who are able to enrol support for the technologies by providing 'visions' of their place in the order of things. He notes Pinch and Bijker's observation that when radically new technologies are introduced, we are likely to see a number of competing visions, networks, and technologies (Pinch and Bijker, 1984). The outcome of these earlier stages of visioning and the search for social support often produces a period of social shaping of technology when a single sociotechnical network stabilizes and becomes dominant. We can see the action of contemporary entrepreneurs in the biotech industry as builders of these sociotechnincal networks, much like Thomas Edison and previous generations of 'inventors'. A recent feature in the business magazine *Canadian Business* illustrates this well. Reviewing the prospects for the biotech companies with a series of articles on the 'biotech bonanza', one article plots the prospects for discovery of the 'holy grail' of a vaccine for Group A streptococcus, which, in the age of antibiotic resistance, is an emerging health risk and a potentially hugely profitable market (Robin, 2001). Biotech company partnerships with the scientific establishment are an important aspect of building business. In a feature on the young entrepreneur Boris Chabursky, head of the Canadian biotech and consulting firm Strategic Health Innovations, his strategy for building his private-sector network is quoted:

The key is, we try to talk to everyone – analysts, investment bankers and venture caps, academia and private-sector partners – to find out where the opportunities are, where they're not, and who's got the resources start-ups need. Then we connect the dots.

(Staples, 2001: 47)

In the business of technological innovation such practitioners know (like the sociologists of technology) that sociotechnical networks need to be built, and maintained and supported, with particular visions.

Technologies, then, appear capable of introducing elements of fixity to technical-social networks or systems. They carry with them imperatives for action and for establishing or maintaining particular sets of relationships. It is useful to consider how genetic knowledge and technology perform within this network of actants currently constituting the field of public health. We can usefully see public health as a sociotechnical network in process: a field typified by competing visions, competing networks and competing technologies. Currently a new technology is being introduced to the field of medicine and public health that carries with it great rhetorical power. It promises to transform this network of actors by introducing innovation. The new genetic knowledge and techniques carry with them an imperative for change, and an imperative that suggests the need to establish new sets of relationships between key actors in the field – particularly between the state, the professions, industrial corporations, communities and citizens. Newer approaches to the study of technology can help us understand and make sense of the current changes in the field. To illustrate this point we must first examine the network of public health.

The field of public health

The birth of public health is not easy to date, but we can say that domain specificity in relation to health – 'public', 'personal' or 'private' – is a fairly recent preoccupation. It has occurred only in the last three hundred years or so as part of the rise of modern biotechnical and scientific knowledge. Not all health strategy has specified public and private spheres. Early systems of thought, such as those codified by Galen, linked health to the flows of humours, which were themselves intimately linked to the forces of the seasons and the movement of the universe. Entirely different metaphysical notions of personal health existed, in which the movement of the cosmos was directly related to our 'internal' health. The moon and the sun were integral parts of the system of elements and forces that made up the substance of our bodies, and embodied existence was not as easily separated from the rest of the universe. In early Greek and Roman thought, however, there existed what appear to be precursors to the distinctions now routinely made between public and personal health. Ancient medicine accounted for the role of personal regimens and diet in warding off disease. Galen's classification of the 'natural' (innate constitutional), the 'non-natural' (environmental) and the preternatural (pathological) causes of health and disease allowed advice to be given on the intake of air, food and drink as well as motion rest, sleep and accidents of the soul (Porter, 1997). Moreover, the Hippocratic notions of 'endemic' (always present) and 'epidemic' (occasional and excessive) disease are direct ancestors of the concepts used in contemporary public health and epidemiology.

In ancient times and throughout the Middle Ages in Europe isolation was seen as an appropriate way of regulating those diseases perceived to be spread by contact. The use of the *cordon sanitaire* in seventeenth century Europe, with its roots in the much older institution of the lazaretto or 'pest house', became an institutionalized strategy foreshadowing later developments in the government of the health of populations. The newer preventive methods of sanitation and immobilization suited the developing discourses of enlightenment and liberalism (Porter, 1997). Contemporary concepts of public health would appear to owe much to the early modern period.

Definitions of public health often seem elusive and differ across professional cultures and decades. While many practitioners in the West date public health to the first UK public health act of 1848, they also acknowledge conceptual developments in Germany and France at that time. The early development of the field was associated with the health problems of newly industrialized cities in northern Europe much earlier. Health in the public sphere can be related to the idea of social medicine, which has been intimately tied to the development of greater state intervention under the doctrine of mercantilism. The early history of public health is linked to the ideas of social medicine, health administration, medical policing (*Medizinalpolizei*) and social reform (Rosen, 1958); more recent attempts at definition have tried to account for public health as a field of knowledge. Frenk (1993) argues that the discipline (or perhaps more accurately field of study) of public health has constructed two major objects of analysis: the epidemiological study of the health conditions of populations, and the study of the organized social responses to these conditions. These foci correspond to two older lines of thought with their roots in the worship of Hygeia and Aesculapius (Dubos, 1959). They provide a taxonomy and an analytical focus, which subdivides health research into biomedical research (the subindividual level), clinical research (individual level) and public health research (population level). Frenk's taxonomy defines public health not only as a field of enquiry but also as a space for professional practice. His notion of public health attempts to be comprehensive and holistic and, as 'an arena for action, the modern conception of public health goes beyond fragmentary dichotomies, such as personal versus environmental services, preventive versus curative activities, and public versus private responsibilities.... In this sense the essence of public health is the health of the public.' (Frenk, 1993: 477).

Frenk (1993) has argued that historically the practice of public health usually has five separate connotations. The adjective 'public' normally refers to government action in the public sector, which distinguishes it from general medicine and other fields of health study and practice, as it did from the 'private' concerns of health at its inception. Public approximates to the dictionary definition of that which affects, or is for the benefit of, the people as a whole, the community or the state. Frenk's second element specifies some notion of participation of the organized community. A third element relies on the definition by exclusion of that which is not public health – personalized health. The notion of 'non-personalized' relies on a distinction between domains. The development of public health emerged as an area distinct from hospital-based practice, which was the focus of the clinic, with its own distinct history (Foucault, 1976). The work of late eighteenth and early nineteenth century figures such as the German Johan Peter Frank and Jules Guerin in France was important in identifying the social realm as one in which health interventions should be targeted. Indeed diligent statistical data-gathering work in France and the UK was to form the basis of not simply medical sciences, but also social science and the study of 'the social' (Foucault, 1980). Reformers of the mid-nineteenth century such as Virchow in Germany and Chadwick in the UK were to link medical science and political transformation to attack the social roots of typhus and other epidemics. Such reformers argued that only socioeconomic and political means alongside medical interventions could improve the health of populations. The linking of health to radical social reform was to become more limited in late nineteenth century Europe. However, the idea of 'social medicine' had established health as a social good that governments were to safeguard for the common good. 'Social medicine depended on scientifically informed technocratically determined actions by the state' (Porter and Porter, 1988: 102). It is possibly because intervention technology in public health was essentially social and political that the field has remained so resistant to easy definition. The first edition of the *Oxford Textbook of Public Health* (Holland *et al.*, 1984), for example, goes to some lengths to avoid a single definition of public health and opts instead to 'portray the philosophy and underlying principles of the practice of public health' (Preface; Holland *et al.*, 1984).

We are often left with operationalized definitions, of which Winslow's is one of the most frequently quoted and possibly one of the most general:

> Public health is the science and the art of preventing disease, prolonging life, and promoting physical (and mental) health and efficiency through organised community efforts for the sanitation of the environment, the control of community infections, and education of the individual in principles of personal hygiene, the organization of medical and nursing service for the early diagnosis and treatment of disease, and the development of the social machinery which will ensure to every individual in the community a standard of living adequate for the maintenance of health.
>
> (Winslow, 1920: 309)

These foci are common in Frenk's distinction between the academic study and the field of practice. With such a broad focus, the field of public health may be subject to change by one element or another, such as the introduction of a new technique. The development of knowledge on the transmission of water borne infection in the mid-nineteenth century, and the subsequent technologies of sewerage and sanitation, are examples of how technological change in one aspect of public health influences the field as a whole. In these cases the emphasis shifted towards structural environmental intervention.

Definitions of public health as a field of study, then, are varied but contain some common elements. Featuring in such definitions are key foci, including the triumvirate: the individual (or host), the environment (or context) and the agent (or contagion). These have sometimes been rephrased as people, products and place (WHO, The World Health Organization, 1988). Definitions also contain a common concern with intervention through social and behavioural techniques in the management of populations. Finally, public health usually also refers to a series of preventive services – a separate subsystem of services provided by the state and parallel to the mainstream of high-technology curative medicine (Frenk, 1993: 472). This group of preventive services determines how the host, environment and agent are acted upon, and how that action will determine the shape of those services. Current practice is still intimately concerned with the conception of environment, agent and host. Changes in the understanding of each of these concepts will have a bearing on the field as a whole.

In the next section we examine some of the ways in which the new genetics as a form of technology and knowledge is entering the sociotechnical network of public health defined above. These forms of knowledge, technique and technology are still new, and their impact on the network is still in development and far from stabilized. Competing visions and networks as well as technologies, are causing turbulence. We illustrate this by discussing some of the ways in which the new genetic knowledge and techniques are beginning to be considered in relation to the understanding of three fundamental elements of pubic health: the host, the environment and the agent. The new knowledge and technology are attempting to reconfigure the current understanding of host, agent and environment. During this period of turbulence the certainties provided by the relatively fixed conceptions of the objects of the field are being questioned, developed and opened up to critical reflection. We will examine the three elements in turn.

The host

Understanding of the host in public health is couched in concerns for the individual subject and for populations. The major part of this book is concerned with changing conceptions of the host and the population that are being engendered by the arrival of the 'new genetics'. New genetic knowledge and technologies are introducing elements of apparent 'personal' choice and responsibility into areas of life that have previously been considered 'public' concerns. Such change has implications for the ways that health care is being organized at the turn of the century. Conceptions of the host are central to wider public-health discourse, and the arrival of the new genetics appears to have far-reaching consequences for this concept also.

The subject of public health has changed over time. Armstrong (1995) has noted the ways in which the gaze of public health has been extended throughout the nineteenth and twentieth centuries. The behaviour of the host, or individual, became a focus of public health discourse at the turn of the twentieth century, for example, as authorities attempted to instil self-discipline and 'temperance' in the use of alcohol and other recreational drugs. Individuals and groups of potential 'addicts' were identified for treatment and prevention (Harrison, 1971). By the late twentieth century a different understanding of drug problems had emerged in which all citizens were expected to monitor and regulate their own, and other people's, drug use to reduce the risks of substance misuse (Bunton, 2001; Levine, 1978). These changes in understanding of the host and populations reflected changing social values and forms of governance. Conceptions of the host in health and public health discourse reproduce particular understandings or versions of the body. In this sense the body is not a fixed physical state but changes according to social and historical circumstance. We are reminded at this point of Turner's functionalist question 'What types of bodies do societies want?' (Turner, 1992), suggestive of a particular approach to understanding the historically specific body.

Recent work in the human sciences has portrayed both subjectivity and our experiences of our bodies as far more fluid than would be assumed from the 'naturalistic' accounts in biomedical science (Lupton, 2000). Experience of the body varies across time, space and culture. An increased flexibility of bodies and selves is said to be a defining feature of late-modern existence (Giddens, 1991, 1999). The study of the sociology of the body has demonstrated that, far from being transparent to the gaze of medical science, the 'truth' of bodies is generated within social processes and reflects social relations of power. Bodies are always contingent and specific to historical and social location. The work of Michel Foucault was pivotal in pointing to the various ways in which the body became the object of the clinical gaze from the late eighteenth century onwards. The modern body, constructed in secular scientific discourse, was not the same as that of a few centuries earlier. That idea of the body was the outcome of a different knowledge and power, largely related to religious understanding of the place of the flesh in the order of the universe (Mellor and Shilling, 1997). Feminist analysts have also been important in highlighting the social relativity of the body and its production within patriarchal power relations. The female body constructed as frail, volatile, 'leaky' or problematic reproduces and maintains women's subordination and tries to make this position appear natural and justifiable (Shildrick, 1997).

Sociologists and epidemiologists have tended to conceive of bodies as profoundly social products, and socially mutable. The vast literature studying the social inequalities of health illustrates how morb-idity and mortality are products of social location. Epidemiologists seem to be acknowledging the existence of more 'flexible' forms of subjectivity and embodiment in recent years (Krieger, 1999). Different social location produces different morphology. These differences are not simply the outcome of the differential access of social groups (related to class, ethnicity or gender) to different physical environments but also to experience of the social fabric itself – to different types of social cohesion or social capital (Wilkinson, 1996).

Disciplines adopting a social understanding of the body have provided a critique of medical science and its tendency to reproduce a naïve universal version of the body and the population. The recent work on genetics also appears to challenge this position. Developments in microbiology and genetics have rendered notions of the body and population as dynamic and fluid as previous versions of the socially produced body. Although reproduced by technological means not social processes, the geneticized body is a plastic body, open to change, development and improvement. The socially generated ideals of perfection can, so the visionaries predict, be realized through the use of genetic science. For public health these changing notions of the host present some fundamental challenges. The public health field currently holds on to two ideas of the body, as both a medically universal and a socially produced body. It has seemed able to hold on to a relativist and a universal notion of the body at the same time. The new genetics exposes this contradiction.

There are differences between social accounts of the body and geneticized accounts, however, which relate to the levels of complexity in the role of the social determination of the body. While accounts of the social generation of the body acknowledge considerable complexity in the nature and sites of its construction (often taking into account interactions between biotic and social systems), many geneticized accounts of the body and the population tend to be simplistic or reductionist in nature. Petersen (1998a) has noted the reductionist pursuit of perfection in much of the recent literature in relation to public health. Elsewhere a number of authors have documented this reductionist tendency in recent literature (Nelkin and Andrews, 1999). These accounts are described in more detail in Chapter 4. In part, this reductionism may be seen as the result of exaggeration and rhetorical force added to many accounts because of their 'visioning' quality. New geneticists have entered the arena of public health advocating new technological innovation and are currently involved in attempting to build a network and enlisting social support for their cause. The case is often overstated. Such 'visioning' often accompanies the building of a technosocial network (or in this case the rebuilding of the technosocial network of public health). These accounts revise the nature of the host and, as Kerr and Cunningham-Burley (2000) have pointed out, redefine the nature of 'the social'

Conceptions of the mutable social body apparent in social and epidemiological treatments of the host adopt an expansive notion of 'the social' and the role it plays in determining the body. This conception is more akin to traditional notions of the social to be found in public health and its concerns with the industrial environment. Reductive accounts of the geneticized body present a very restricted notion of the social. They redraw the boundaries of the social in ways that afford little determining power over health, and therefore give little reason for intervention by social programmes of public health.

The 'new' genetics presents a vision of increased choice 'empowerment', as is outlined in Chapter 2. We can find utopian and dystopian visions in such accounts, which are indicative of the changing understanding of human agency and the body. A critique has been developed of the apparent 'shrinking' of social concerns in some genetic reductionist accounts.

In an article titled 'The new eugenics: the case against genetically modified humans', Marcy Darnovsky (2001) comments on the overzealous promotion of a new bioengineered utopia by scientists and pundits who envisage a world in which parents will strive to afford the latest genetic 'improvements' for their children. The exercise of consumer preferences for offspring options will be the prelude to the technological control of human evolution. Darnovsky quotes the Princeton geneticist and techno-eugenic enthusiast Lee M. Silver, who envisions a future in which affluent parents are 'as likely to arrange genetic enhancements for their children as to send them to private school', and to reproduce in fertility clinics to create an embryo, then to select the physical, cognitive, and behavioural traits they desire for their child-to-be. Silver's book *Remaking Eden: Cloning and Beyond in a Brave New World* (Silver, 1998) is aimed at a lay audience and presents a renewed eugenic population plan based around American consumer choice. Silver predicts the bifurcation of society over time into different genetic social classes, and subsequently into different species. By the year 2350:

> The GenRich – who account for 10 percent of the American population – all carry synthetic genes. Genes that were created in the laboratory.... The GenRich are a modern-day hereditary class of genetic aristocrats.... All aspects of the economy, the media, the entertainment industry, and the knowledge industry are controlled by members of the GenRich class. In contrast, naturals work as low-paid service providers or as laborers.
>
> (Silver, 1998: 3 and 4)

The genetic divide is genetically engineered.

> [A]s time passes ... the GenRich class and the Natural class will become the GenRich humans and the Natural humans – entirely separate species with no ability to cross-breed, and with as much romantic interest in each other as a current human would have for a chimpanzee.
>
> (Silver, 1998: 4)

Individualized market choice may have some serious consequences for the organization of the class structure, via such germ line engineering. What for Silver is an inevitable if not desirable future, appears to Darnovsky (and perhaps to us) as a dystopian vision. The threat of the creation of a genetic underclass and other unpalatable futures has mobilized opposition, for example in the form of the Council for Responsible Genetics (http://www.gene-watch.org) and the Campaign Against Human Genetic Engineering (http://www.users.globalnet.co.uk/~cahge). Such an extreme techno-eugenic vision of the future relies on methods of selective reproduction and would appear to be far from the proposed measured practices of public health which are currently advocated.

Such hyperbole is difficult to evaluate and may be seen as a provocative overstatement of the case, typical of 'visioning' work, that attempts to summon support and build sociotechnical networks. These texts may be considered as rhetorical devices to support this process and are not, we may surmise, attempting to match the rigour of scientific argument. As rhetoric or popular accounts of science, however, these visionary statements reproduce a 'modernist', reductive, technologically determined vision of the universe that is rendered controllable by the progress of science (Kerr and Cunningham-Burley, 2000). They bolster beliefs in the possibility of the technological determination of the world. Choice' over bodily form and personal biography, it is suggested, increases as we are released from traditional ties, systems of belief and social relationships. Life increasingly becomes a planning process, and an individualized one at that (Beck-Gernsheim, 1996).

> A human being is becoming his or her own project right down to organising, distinguishing features, genes. ... Someone who knows his or her genetic susceptibilities, his or her particular risk factors, can prepare him or herself for them, perhaps avert fate – prevent the onset of an illness, secure a longer life for him or herself.
>
> (Beck-Gernsheim, 1996: 141)

Public health's moral authority is implicated in social regulation and governance. Like other medico-scientific discourses, it 'constructs' as well as analyses its subject of enquiry. It is in this sense that Michel Foucault spoke of modern scientific thought as being intimately concerned with the production of the modern subject. The science of epidemiology, for example, continues to construct particular groups and populations within the broader values of the Western world (Lupton, 1995). Certain groups and bodies continue to be catego-rized as troublesome, frail or problematic, such as those of women

(Martin, 1994; Shildrick, 1997), homosexuals (Waldby, 1996) or black people (Nazroo, 1998). These forms of knowledge influence self-knowledge and self-formation. As well as providing psychological and experiential forms of self-knowing, through potential genetic manipulation and 'choice', contemporary science also provides techniques for what might be referred to as the 'biological' body. It is in this sense that Foucault (1980) wrote of modern science's involvement in modern forms of governance by administering 'life' itself. Attending to the biological needs of the population as a living species was a defining moment in modern concepts of government (Foucault, 1986). Contemporary public health discourses engender forms of self-regulation and behavioural control in ways that construct prudent risk-managing subjectivities. Health-promoting regimens provide, using Foucault's term, 'techniques of the self' that create the modern individual as a self-manager of health and risk, to suit contemporary forms of governance.

The visioning accounts of writers and actors such as Silver are not the only narratives emerging from microbiology, however. A number of different visions are available, presenting different versions of the body or the host and its determinants. High profile, amply funded genetic research can often eclipse other scientific work in the field. Whilst reductive media portrayals of developments, as we will see in Chapter 4, have tended to foreground 'heroic' discoveries, technological achievements and future promise, they tend to neglect, as popular accounts of science often do, the subtlety, controversy and internal inconsistency in the field. Other versions of science and the host suggest a different role for genetic and social technologies in public health.

Some recent critiques of genetic reductionism, or the 'extended theory of the gene', have come from cell and molecular biologists, with calls for a substantial qualification of the genetic component in understanding health and disease. Reviewing such critical work, Strohman (2000) argues that whilst knowledge of genetics can be argued to be *essential* to causal accounts of organisms' phenotype and the development of most diseases, it is not a *sufficient* explanation. An adequate explanation of disease must also look to other forms of biological regulation that are developmental, complex and open to environmental influence.

Attempts by gene cloners, armed with advanced statistical devices, to redefine common polygenic diseases in terms of genetic tendency and attempts by behavioural scholars of various backgrounds to apply monogenic 'software' to the reality of polygenic human traits all appear to discount the warnings coming from cell molecular embryological studies that genetic approaches alone are not sufficient to yield a satisfactory picture of complex phenotypes.

We have wrongly extended the theory of the gene to another area altogether: we have been lulled into reasoning that if the gene theory works at one level, from DNA to protein, it must work at all higher levels as well. We have thus extended the theory of the gene to the realm of gene management. But gene management is an entirely different process involving interactive cellular processes that display a complexity that may be described only as trans-calculational, a mathematical term for 'mind-boggling'.

(Strohman, 2000: 104)

Whilst the simple storybook explanations provide a model of something akin to a 'gene' machine, it is argued that 'the cell is beginning to look more like a complex adaptive system rather than a factory floor of robotic gene machines' (Strohman, 2000: 108). Such accounts describe a more flexible genome that is hardly the 'building block' of life that appears in popular accounts. This multi-levelled physiological analysis counters simple biogenic reductionism.

Strohman identifies three modes of activity and pathways that operate to determine phenotypes in an organism: monogenic, polygenic and epigenetic. Monogenic pathways specify one gene → one trait pathways. Examples of monogenic diseases are sickle cell anaemia and Duchnenne muscular dystrophy. Though open to environmental influence also, monogenic pathways can operate without environmental influence. Polygenic pathways refer to phenotypes that are determined by many genes acting together. Epigenetics implies that interaction between environmental signals and genes is complex and extended, and includes individual organismal experience. In short, the epigenetic interaction pathway implies greater complexity of interaction. Epigenesis is defined in the following account:

Classical genetics has revealed the mechanism for the transmission of genes from generation to generation, but the strategy of the genes in unfolding the developmental programme remains obscure. Epigenetics comprises the study of the mechanisms that impart temporal and spatial control on the activity of all those genes required for the development of a complex organism from the zygote to the adult.

(Holiday, 1990: 330)

Such definitions establish a level of control above the genome, but at levels of complexity that challenge, if not evade, theoretical insight (Strohman, 2000; Webster and Goodwin, 1997). Controls may be found at many levels in the organism, and all levels are open to environmental influence, epigenetic networks, skeletal membrane units and networks of cells.

This analysis would cast some doubt upon the usefulness of phrases such as 'the genetic' basis of disease. It suggests that complex physiological, polygenic disease and growth regulation are not linear in process and require a non-linear alternative methodology that can capture the complexity of adaptive, unpredictable systems. Such an analysis might suggest a far more modest role for genetics in developing an understanding of public health. It relies on a more complex understanding of the host and its relationship to the environment. It appears to challenge reductive, simplistic understandings of these things.

A similar, more qualified role for public health is apparent in a recent collection of public health readings by Zimmern (1999), who makes the case for public health's response to recent developments in biochemistry and states that:

The public health agenda has to date been influenced almost entirely by a consideration of the environmental influences on health. These influences remain important and a continued momentum on health promotion interventions directed at the external environment will be essential for the public health function. Nevertheless, insights generated from molecular biology and genetic studies require that we now attend to and explore the complexities of the interaction between genetic and environmental factors, that we regard the interaction between nature and nurture as complementary rather than competing explanations, and that we attempt to promote health and prevent disease by having regard to how environmental factors and human behaviour might have differential effects on disease risk by virtue of the genetic susceptibility of particular individuals.

Genetic mechanisms influence the prevalence of disease and ill health, and must be considered in establishing population-based policies and public health action in much the same way as they have been in the treatment of individual patients.

(Zimmern, 1999: 136)

He goes on to argue that evolutionary mechanisms, such as natural and social selection processes, are now apparent to biologists, who are more sophisticated than, and avoid the simple biological determinism of, the morally tainted eugenics movement, claiming:

The interaction of genes and environment has been well established at the level of the cell and its biochemical pathways; similar interactions take place at the population level, where the differential sensitivities of diverse populations in society to environmental influences are progressively exposed.

(Zimmern, 1999: 136)

Zimmern distinguishes between 'genotypic' intervention strategies, such as the selective termination of pregnancy and pre-implantation diagnosis and the selective destruction of embryos (which has connotations of eugenics); and 'phenotypic' interventions, which rely on 'selective environmental manipulation for susceptible subgroups in the population' (1999: 137). Ironically, even phenotypic intervention calls for more individualizing attention to be drawn to genetic risk. Zimmern quotes the example of genes responsible for the metabolism of drugs and environmental toxins. Some individuals are genetically fast or slow to metabolize, or have a greater lung cancer risk. Genetic susceptibility to ultraviolet rays has also been identified. The number of 'phenotypic' examples is small. However, it points the way towards a more rigorous division of the population and more specific application of health regimens.

The former 'genotypic' mechanisms have, perhaps, received more attention in public debate and recent research. Silver's techno-eugenic vision of the future provides a rather crude rendering of the potential for reproductive control, but it points to two important implications of the new genetics for public health: the individualization of risk, and the flexibility of the body. A feature of the techno-eugenic thinking is the assumption of a more complex, flexible form of host. Individual bodies and populations are being reconfigured, and the subject of public health in the age of new genetics and biotechnology is one that is open to manipulation and adjustment. Not only is the genetic body open to manipulation across generations, it is also open to therapeutic intervention more directly by somatic therapeutic techniques aimed not only at the human embryo but also at 'faulty' adult cell and organ regeneration (Martin, 1995; Spallone, 1992). The genetically modified body is, in this sense, a cyborg, a hybrid part human part technology. Such melding of technology and humanity is considered problematic, if not abhorrent, in Western cultures, despite the many positive health and social benefits that may accrue from being 'monsters'. Donna Haraway (1991) has welcomed human machine hybridity and the 'promise' it offers humanity. Elsewhere, Sobchack (1995) has documented the oneness of prosthetic limbs, and the affection one can accord to such body extensions. Cochlear implants, pacemakers and a range of other technologies have extended the human body in one way or another. The genetically modified body may be seen as another area in which the human body can be modified and 'improved' by technology. It represents another way in which the host of public health is being destabilized, changed and perhaps even strengthened. Recombinant humans may be built to be stronger in the face of hostile agents and environments than their 'natural' counterparts.

The 'new genetic' science, then, erodes traditional assumptions of a stable 'biological' body in a similar manner to social science treatments of the body or host. Visions and counter-visions are being presented. 'Strong' programmes exist which assume a larger place for the new genetic techniques in determining health. These exist alongside 'weaker' programmes which qualify the possible contributions to be made by these new technologies and integrate them with expansive social techniques in public health programme design. There are differing visions of the possibilities for determining the host of public health. 'Stronger' visions allow less space for social and environmental determination or influence of the host, and thus threaten some fundamental assumptions within public health (Willis, 1998). 'Weaker' visions provide more interactive models of environmental determination of the host. Estimation of the determining effect of the environment is dependent upon the way that environments are conceived. Here, too, the newer genetic technologies are implicated in changing the understanding of nature and the environment, with implications for public health. We now turn briefly to consider such change.

Environment

The environment is fundamental to concepts of health in general but is usually seen as the special preserve of public health medicine. A concern with Air, Water and Places can be traced to Hippocrates and Greek thought, and later to Roman medicine (Kitto, 1957). The environment is so much a cornerstone of public health that the date of birth of the discipline (1848) relates to the heyday of major improvements in the hazardous environments of the early industrial period. Victorian sanitary reforms aimed at reducing the spread of infectious disease in many ways define the 'classical' period of public health. The publication of Chadwick's report *Sanitary Conditions of the Labouring Population of Great Britain* in 1842, with its meticulous research and documentation, was to set the terms of debate about the relationship between the physical environment and disease for the following decades and underscored momentous public health reform (Baggot, 2000). Use of the term physical environment is important here. Physical approximates to the dictionary definition 'of or pertaining to material nature ... or matter' (Little *et al.*, 1973) public health focus but with a slightly different, expanded notion of the environment, and one that emphasizes the human as opposed to the natural environment.

The environment received increased public health attention in the later decades of the twentieth century. In the early 1990s Draper (P. Draper, 1991) argued for a 'new' approach to public health that was 'green sensitive' and recognized that the human-made environments in rich and poor countries could adversely affect people's health. The 'core' of public health, he claimed, should be environmental in focus, taking in the physical and the social and economic aspects of existence – the 'total environment' (P. Draper, 1991: 10). Whilst this definition of public health includes the more common practices of screening and specialist public interventions such as behaviour change, it placed importance on the role of healthy public policy generation in the building of sustainable environmental policy. Milio's definition captured the sentiments of the time by defining healthy public policy as:

'Ecological in perspective, multi-sectoral in scope and participatory in strategy' (Milio, 1986). The Third International Conference on Health Promotion of the WHO, held in 1991 in Sundsvall, Sweden, on 'Supportive Environments for Health', attempted to fuse the focus on health, the environment and sustainable development (WHO, 1991). This followed on from a number of international developments that appeared to embrace environmentalist issues.

At the end of the last century calls were made to make public health more responsible for countering potentially hostile, socioeconomic environments, which in many ways reflected the preoccupation of nineteenth century public health activists. The interest was in building a social medicine and welfare state to counter the worst effects of rapid industrial development and the environmental damage it created. Whilst Zimmern (quoted above) argues that the environmental aspects of public health have been a focus for too long, others claim that the environment has been relatively neglected. One reason for this is that authors such as Draper were drawing upon a broader definition of environment than is common in public health discourse, which includes social as well as physical features. Such thinking draws upon international studies of the environment such as the World Commission on Environment and Development (the Brundtland Report, 1987), and the *State of the World* reportsz coming from the Worldwatch Institute. Environmental issues climbed the public health policy agenda in the late twentieth century. The 1992 Rio Earth Summit focused world attention upon the limits of endless technologico-economic development. Sustainable development became a concern, as well as possibilities for 'Ecological Modernisation' (Hajer, 1995). Environmentalist public health builds upon nineteenth century public health concerns in an attempt to tackle hazards of the physical environment, for example sewerage and clean water supply. The 'New Public Health' which emerged in the early 1980s also included a socioeconomic environment such as unemployment. Draper's account continues to consider the environment as a product of public policies such as those determining levels of employment, energy policy trends, economic policy (such as the production of tobacco), the arms trade and macroeconomic policies on issues such as Third World debt. A distinction is maintained between the natural and the human or 'man-made' environment. In attempting to bring the social, economic and political back into public health, however, the argument often glosses over difficulties faced when trying to separate the 'natural' from the human-made environment.

Though it is central to their concerns, the advocates of a 'new' public health remain remarkably unreflective about the nature of the environment. Problems with definition have been noted, particularly the environment's tendency to include everything (Hannigan, 1995). Although WHO (1997) has stated that 25 per cent of preventable ill health is due to poor environment, defining how environment affects health remains problematic (Baggot, 2000). Whilst expanding the entity of the environment to include the human and non-natural environment, little attention is given to the issue of how we demarcate the two or, in fact, how we define the environment at all. Such lack of specificity is not possible when we consider the place of the 'new' genetics in relation to the environment, and reflection on the phenomena of the environment is unavoidable. Other disciplines, such as sociology and social policy, have considered elements of the environment in recent years and are of interest here.

Much recent sociology has noted the socially constructed nature of the environment. Like the related concept – nature – environment is seen as a site for a range of definitional and contestatory activities, often in the global context (Hannigan, 1995). Environmental issues cohere around intersecting and competing social and cultural definitions and interests. Environmental threats involve a range of parties, including private industry, government, regulators, scientists, environmental groups, trade and professional groups and grassroots communities and 'victims'. Environment and environmental risks are the outcome of a range of actors in an increasingly uncertain world of risk calculation and management (Beck, 1992). The onset of 'risk society' would seem to herald a world in which the above groups negotiate to construct levels of consensus and conflict over the risky environments. Complex social and economic processes frequently leave the world a contingent, hazardous and erratic place to live (Bauman, 1997). The increased centrality of science and technology in late modern production practices has, it is argued, produced more human-made hazards and risks, which bring into question the independence of the scientific enterprise (Beck, 1992). Climatic change and nuclear fall-out are seen as the result of human endeavour. A number of threats to the environment emanate from biotechnologies and the new genetics, which directly reflect such concerns.

The arrival of new bio- and genetic technologies and their use represent a significant increase in potential for human manipulation of the environment. The environment and the host may both be manipulated. Increased control of aspects of genetic structure has introduced a range of potential 'environmental risks', the extent of which is determined by negotiation and contestation between interested parties. Introducing changes to the raw materials of industrial production, patterns of labour, health, energy and food production, biotechnologies will dramatically adjust our environments. Genetically altered microorganisms pose potential health risks to humans and animals. Genetically engineered biopesticides and seeds are considered the most lucrative new products of agricultural biotechnology and the new knowledge-rich global economy (discussed in more detail in Chapter 6).

As a branch of the science of biotechnology, genetic modification techniques have the potential to manipulate and refashion nature according to the logic of the marketplace. Because of this, biotechnologies provide opportunities for the development and restructuring of the food system for profit (Bainbridge *et al.*, 2000). The potential 'gene revolution' follows closely on the heels of the 'green revolution' of the agricultural economies in the middle of the last century (Spallone, 1992). This revolution has far-reaching consequences for the environment. Direct environmental manipulation and improvement for public health become a possibility, as do (simultaneously) harmful health effects resulting from this manipulation – either directly or indirectly.

Critics of the use of GM foods have, for instance, shown concern for the long-term impact of new genetic variants on the environment (Mendelson, 1998; Nottingham, 1998). Symbolic attacks on GM products have headline phrases such as 'Frankenfoods' and 'Farmageddon'. Discussions of the dangers to wildlife and biodiversity have been noted, as well as the cross-pollination to neighbouring crops. In addition to the possible direct effects on the human body, hybrid plants could affect resistance to antibiotics and pesticides. Critics of GM technology include consumer groups, grain importers from the European Union countries, organic farmers, environmentalists, scientists, ethicists and religious rights groups, food and advocacy groups, some politicians and trade protectionists.

Their health concerns include fear for the alteration and depletion of the nutritional quality of foods, potential toxicity, possible antibiotic resistance from GM crops, potential allergies and carcinogenicity from consuming GM foods (Uzogara, 2000). More general concerns relate to environmental pollution, unintended gene transfer to wild plants, possible creation of new viruses, toxins and 'super weeds' which will have detrimental effects on wildlife and the wider environment. In addition there is a fear of multinational-led limitation of access to seeds by means of gene patenting and the creation of 'terminator seeds' (Warwick, 2000). These concerns have resulted in the development of procedures of risk judgement and assessment in national governments, such as those of the UK Advisory Committee on Novel Foods and Products (Burke, 2000). The risk of the unknown lies behind many of these considerations. There are fears of an exaggerated North–South global formation resulting from concentration of agricultural power in the hands of multinational companies (Galhardi, 1995). There are also concerns that the wealthier nations will no longer need to import staples such as vanilla, cocoa, coffee, Basmati rice and other crops from poorer predominantly tropical countries. Such fears have resulted in many GM products being seen as high risk and in need of regulation and control (Gaskell *et al.*, 1999).

Consumer resistance in Europe has been so vociferous that a moratorium was placed on new approvals for GM crops (Hileman, 1999). Public opposition in the United States has been less strong and perhaps more open to these newer products (Hoban, 1999). Canada, Australia, Brazil and Argentina have accepted agricultural biotech crops according to the International Service for the Acquisition of Agribiotech Applications (ISAAA). Chinese policy on these developments also seems welcoming of GM products, with 9 per cent of rice production currently being of genetically modified varieties. A referendum in Australia involving 1.2 million people resulted in Australia seeking to become a GM-free zone (Nottingham, 1998). In the UK anti-GM protesters regularly sabotage crops and adopt other means of direct-action protest.

At the heart of much of the fear of GM products is the issue of changing nature to better suit human needs and desires with newer, more radical and untested methods. The voices of protest to GM products illustrate a contrast in approach to reductionist accounts of genetic determinism. These voices draw attention to the unintended consequences of the introduction of newer genetic processes. These consequences are the outcome of complex local conditions. Although the result of the 'neutral' science of genetics, these outcomes have political consequences. There are contrasting episte-mological assumptions at work, which reflect some differences in disciplinary perspective. Adam recently observed that:

> Whilst decontextualized truth continues to play an important role in the physical and mathematical sciences, in the life sciences disembedding plays a far more paradoxical and contentious role. In the field of genotechnology, molecular biologists are divided in their approach to context. Reductionist genetic determinism, for example, is rooted in an understanding that excludes the wider context.
>
> (Adam, 2000: 134)

Much recent research in the new genetics suggests that genes do not work in isolation, that genetic networks are subject to layers of feedback from both the organism's physiology and the relationship to its environment, that feedback can facilitate mutations, and that genes can transfer horizontally, outside the original host organism (Ho *et al.*, 1998; Holdrege, 1996). The isolated facts of genetic knowledge are dependent, then, upon understanding their larger context. Adams points to the importance of time in understanding the processes of the mircroorganism. She quotes Holdrege, who explains that the plant cannot be understood simply in spatial terms but must be seen in time. Over time a plant's processes move beyond their immediate spatial capacity. The controlled laboratory conditions of experimental science, then, with their predictable results, may miss essential elements of environmental actions. Thus, understanding gene technologies in the environment, may require a more environmental focus and one accounting for context.

An interesting feature of recent ecological sociology is that it outlines the semi-independence and value of both the environment and technology. There is a holistic assessment of the role of human endeavour in the development of the environment and human society in general. Less 'anthropocentric' in style, a new ecological paradigm emerged in sociology from the 1970s onwards which adopted a more 'ecocentric' approach in which human endeavour was only one part in a complex web of actors (Buttel, 1999; Dunlop and Catton, 1992/3). Leopold (1966) took the 'biotic community membership' as his starting point. The emphasis here is on an ethical and epistemological stance, which values the connectednesss and interdependence of nature, species and societies. This move involves a shift from thinking of ourselves as members of human society and conquerors of the land to seeing ourselves as 'plain members and citizens of it' (1966: 240). This position bears similarities to one associated with various 'eco-feminists' (Cuomo, 1998), which rejects many aspects of human-centred culture and the rights of sentient individuals, and instead asserts the value of ecosystems. The value of ecological communities is inherent and not reducible to their use value for humans. Such thinking is suggestive of the newer public health ethic suggested by Draper, discussed above. Environmental sociology has described the environment as a site of intersecting social and cultural definitions and interests (Hannigen, 1995). The fact that concepts such as the environment and nature are open to competing definitions creates problems for those organizing 'life-politics'. There is some evidence of a coming together of a range of environmental movement activists under a more widespread politics of nature as a broad social movement (Dobson and Lucardie, 1993; Melucci, 1989; Sutton, 1999). However, the movement highlights some of the difficulties of the concept of nature and environment. It is interesting to note that opponents of GM products have attempted to denigrate the introduction of 'non-natural' phenomena, whilst biotech companies and those in favour of the development of GMO's have emphasized the history of human intervention with nature and the 'naturalness' of this enterprise.

Developments in genetic technologies make us more aware of the increasingly manufactured nature of the 'natural environment'. The division between external/natural and non-external/human environment threat is not easily maintained and cannot simply be factored in, as do some recent accounts of the Environmental Genome Project which attempt to study gene–environment interactions in this way (Brookbank, 1999). Genetically modified tomatoes provide a good example of the reflection on these not so 'natural' processes. Genetically modified tomato paste was the target of much European concern in recent years. Yet the tomato in question is far from that originating in 'nature'. Originally cultivated from the wild in the Andes by the Aztecs, the tomato came to Europe after substantial modification by traditional methods of breeding. When Novartis, the agrochemical and biotech company, developed the new variety, they returned to the Andes to seek disease-resistant varieties to cross with contemporary commercial hybrids (Harvey,

1999). A further transformation of cultivated nature took place in this case in a complex bio-socioeconomic process.

Introduction of modified species alongside 'naturally occurring' host populations, resulting in recombinant or hybrid species, will mean that the distinctions between 'natural' and non-natural in the environment will have little meaning. Whilst many features of the natural environment are produced or at least profoundly influenced by human endeavour, the scale of genetic production and influence over the environment is predicted to be significantly greater than that of previous technological accomplishments. Whilst this shift makes it a significant topic of public health concern and risk assessment, it also makes it a conceptually more difficult one. Public health action cannot, as in previous decades and centuries, address the environment as a relatively stable entity. The contemporary genetically modified environment would appear to be potentially more changeable, erratic, hazardous, and contingent than ever before. It is more directly the outcome of human scientific/technical intervention and as such makes intervention more complex. Dealing with the relatively obdurate 'natural' physical environment is a qualitatively different exercise from negotiating the collective fabrication of the contemporary and future genetic environment. The approach needed is likely to be a more system-oriented one and less linear or instrumental in focus, and one that can adequately deal with the increased presence of technology. Concepts of the environment are generated within a sociotechnical network. There are apparent differing visions of the environment in opposing visions of the future. It would appear that some of the heroic narratives of humanity 'conquering' nature with the aid of technology are less common and more problematic in relation to genetics.

In reflecting upon the introduction of new genetics technologies to public health concepts of the environment, then, we can find evidence of competing visions of our future – utopias and dystopias. Competing networks are being built to develop current technologies. The potential levels of complexity GMOs bring into debates about the environment raise more fundamental questions about the nature of the environment itself. Like 'nature', the environment becomes a site for competing definitional and contestatory activities as a part of political activities involving new social movements and groupings organized around 'life-politics' on the one hand and capital on the other. Genetic technologies would appear to be further problematizing the environment for public health. In doing so, they draw attention to the other element of the public health triumvirate – the agent.

Agent

In public health narratives the agent has largely been seen as the villain of the piece and something in need of eradication, modification or regulation. Agents present a technological challenge. Infectious diseases caused by a single agent formed the focus of much of nineteenth century public health endeavour. The relative successes of inoculation, vaccination and eradication have been the subject of a great deal of debate within public health (Mckeown, 1976). Many early strategies aimed at eliminating harmful agents involved environmental design strategies which attacked the breeding grounds of harmful hosts, such as sewerage, drains and urban and housing design. Eradication of mosquito beds to combat malaria is an example of such approaches. More recently, harmful agents have included consumer products such as tobacco, alcohol and recreational drugs (WHO, 1988). Significantly, this literature has redefined the agent as a 'product', and represents a shift away from infectious diseases towards the so-called 'life-style' ailments or diseases of affluence. The new genetic technologies enter considerations of agents in various ways. Genetically modified goods, as we have noted above, may be classed as potentially harmful products themselves and added to the diseases of affluence of the non-infectious realm. Genetic technologies can also be used to attack or assist in the attack of other harmful agents. One area in which genetics has played a part is vaccine development. Though not without its own dangers, vaccination possibilities have been opened up by the capacity for cell manipulation, with mixed success (Spallone, 1992). The use of genetic technologies in combination presents possibilities here.

Recent media reports of a 'vaccine in GM fruit that could wipe out hepatitis B' illustrate something of the possibilities in this area of public health. A story in the UK *Guardian* in 2000 told how tomatoes and bananas could be genetically modified to contain hepatitis B vaccine and thus provide a very inexpensive means of vaccinating whole populations, making total world-wide eradication of hepatitis B (and some other diseases) conceivable. Tomatoes and bananas offer the promise of modern eradication of infectious disease rather like vaccination and inoculation programmes did in the previous two centuries. Professor Arntzen of the Cornell Boyce Thomson Institute for plant research at Cornell University, involved in the trial of this method, claimed:

> We have rid the world of small pox through the vaccination and we are close with polio. Now I believe we can do it with hepatitis B too.
>
> (*Guardian*, 8 September 2000)

The near science-fiction element of genetically engineered potent fruit is brought back to earth and applied to the serious business of modern medicine. The article points out that 'the breakthrough' is seen as a vindication of, and public 'relations saviour' for, the US biotech industry – a way of transforming GM developments into a positive light. The article relies on promises and envisaged developments – virtual further findings, technologies, investment and uptake – that will enable governments to save lives throughout the world. A close reading of this 'breakthrough' reveals that the reports are based on 'successful experiments' and only three clinical trials.

Another way in which the agent can be controlled is by the use of genetic design. The attempt to introduce competing mosquito strains, incapable of carrying harmful malarial larvae is one such example of this (*Guardian*, 15 November 2000). The knock-on effects on the environment of such science are problematic, to say the least. These dangers are similar to those experienced in the 'frontier science' of experimental crop pest eradication (Hatchwell, 1989; Spallone, 1992). Perhaps because the potential problems in this area are great, it remains an under-developed aspect of the genetic contribution to public health.

Elsewhere, Ho and colleagues have painted a less than optimistic picture of the possibilities for genetically engineering away infectious diseases (Ho *et al.*, 1998). World Health Organization reports of an impending crisis caused by re-emerging infectious diseases has fuelled concern about horizontal gene transfer possibilities. As current pathogens are resistant to known treatments, the fear of further resistance must be a concern:

> Many pathogens have crossed species barriers having acquired genes from phylogenetically distant species that are involved in

their ability to cause disease. Recent findings document the extremely wide scope of horizontal gene transfer and the extensive recombination between genetic material from unrelated species that have contributed to the emergence of virulence and antibiotic resistance. The past 15 years coincided with the development of genetic engineering biotechnology on a commercial scale. Genetic engineering depends on designing vectors for cloning and transferring genes and involves artificially recombining and manipulating genes from unrelated species and their viral pathogens, thereby enhancing the probability for horizontal gene transfer and recombination. The urgent question which needs to be addressed is the extent to which genetic engineering biotechnology, by facilitating horizontal gene transfer and recombination, is contributing to the resurgence of infectious, drug resistant diseases. And will continue to do so if allowed to proceed unchecked.

(Ho *et al.*, 1998: 3)

In considering the conception of the agent in pubic health discourse, then, we can identify ways in which the 'new' genetics and recent biotechnology developments are attempting to redefine the host – for the betterment of health or otherwise. Though not without their own iatrogenic risk, such interventions are reconfiguring that which was seen as a relatively stable feature of the world as we know it: threatening contagion. Like previous notions of the environment and the host, the agent appears as an unstable category that defies the contemporary public health gaze. Contemporary genetics, and the ideas of science accompanying it, appear to deconstruct the world as we know it in important ways, along with key concepts of public health. There would appear to be competing visions available in relation to the contribution of new genetic technologies towards treatment of the agent: those that suggest these technologies can help reduce health risk and those that fear they could introduce more health risks.

Genetic technology and public health

It has been argued that we can usefully consider the new genetics as a novel technology developed within sociotechnical systems consisting of multiple actors comprising the public health field. Key actors in this network include the state, private corporations and biotech companies, scientific communities, pressure groups and social movements, environmental and 'life-politics' groups, farming and a number of international policy coordinating bodies. The newer genetic technologies and knowledges, we have argued, are problematizing some of the basic tenets of the public health field, including those relating to the host and the environment. Current geno-technologies and the genetic imagination that accompanies them have resulted in different relationships developing in the classic triumvirate of public health.

The new genetic technologies, like any technology, develop in interaction with sociotechnical networks in interaction with human networks, and do not have the simple determining power often attributed to new technologies. The process of technological development is incomplete. There would appear to be competing visions and networks and actors within the public health field. The network as a whole is not yet stable. Ethical dispute and debate is symptomatic of this turbulence.

In acknowledging the role of technology in the generation of public health problematics, we not only make sense of recent changes in the field brought on by the new genetics but can also make observations about changes in the field in previous periods. With such a broad focus, the field of public health may be subject to change and modification due to developments in the environment, host, agent or technology. Above we noted the changing nature of the environment and the call for a 'new' public health to address the new environmental threats of the late twentieth century. Technological developments within one area of public health, the environment for example, can have implications for the field as a whole. The development of knowledge and techniques for restricting the transmission of water borne infection in the nineteenth century, and the development of technologies of sewerage and sanitation, for example, changed the focus of public health as a whole towards structural and environmental intervention. A contrary shift occurred in the early twentieth century, however, due to technological developments in non-public health medicine, which drew attention away from public health and 'social medicine' and privileged hospital curative medicine. Changing social conditions (Turner, 1992) in turn fostered this technology. A medically dominated, specialist health service grew up in this period which was individually focused and required a fee-for-service general practice, prompted by a growing middle-class demand for health care. This system bolstered the emerging belief in technological medicine. Dominant values of liberalism and individualism fostered 'professional individualism', and the doctor–client relationship was opposed to the social interventionism required by social medicine (Turner, 1992: 132).

Technological advances were to play a support role in these sociopolitical developments. Several major technological advances in science and in medicine were making surgery, treatment and hospital practices safer and more effective. Anaesthesia and germ theory were progressing, as were antiseptic procedures based on the work of Lister and Pasteur. There is a sense in which social medicine and the concerns for public health in the late nineteenth and early twentieth centuries were at odds with the development of scientific or 'technomedicine'. The so called 'golden age' of scientific, technomedicine is normally seen to be in the period 1910 to 1950, a period in which the rising fortunes of the medical profession were instituted in the university systems of Europe and the USA, in increasingly specialized medical education and research institutes along the lines recommended in the influential Flexner Report (1910). This golden age was to substantially influence the development of public health over that period.

Interestingly, developments in microbiology during the same period heralded, for some leading public health progressives, a 'New Public Health' (Porter, 1997). Charles Chapin believed that bacteriology completely differentiated this new public health from its older form. Practitioners appeared to recognize a shift in the paradigm, one which moved away from the environmental focus, just as practitioners such as Draper, Ashton and others in the late twentieth century identified another shift in the paradigm reinstating the importance of environment (albeit a slightly different one). This use of 'new' and 'old' would appear to be a complete reversal of more recent understanding of 'new' and 'old' public health, which has called for a return to the principles of social causation applied in the work of Chadwick (Ashton, 1992). Around the same time, the notion of 'biological regeneration' and notions of inevitable 'biological decline' were making inroads in the UK through the work of the English biomedical statistician Francis Galton. Degenerationist and hereditarian theories gained some momentum in Europe and the USA, challenging much of the legitimacy of public health reform. If preventive medicine were applied, then we might save the weak as well as the strong, it was argued, thereby undermining the 'racial' superiority of superior breeds. Advocating marriage regulation, sequestration of the mentally deficient and sterilization of the unfit, eugenicists throughout Europe and in the colonies of Australia and New Zealand gained some influence in preparing to rid society of its unwanted elements (Porter, 1997). The realities of these ideas were to be acted upon in Germany during the Second World War. They were also to become a part of immigration policy in a number of countries. In the United States compulsory sterilization laws were passed in forty-four states. Belief in eugenics and the place of breeding as the only salvation of 'civilized races' owed much to the paranoia engendered by imperialist ambitions in Western Europe in the late nineteenth and early twentieth centuries. These developments also illustrate the transformations that new knowledges and techniques can produce in our understanding of the tenets of public health.

Recent technological changes introduced by the new genetics may be ushering in another 'new public health' that heralds a new way of conceptualizing the relationship between agent, environment and host. If so, this reconceptualization will affect broader cultural categories including fundamental oppositions such as those between nature and culture, body and technology, the individual and the collective and the public and the private. Public health is part of a dynamic system of interdependencies and is not simply led by a small number of professionals and experts. In such systems human endeavour is only one element in the dynamic interplay between physical objects and technologies.

Conclusion

Whilst constituting an academic discipline or field of study, public health refers to a complex network of relationships, crossing the public and private realms and including the state, citizen and corporate actors. We have highlighted the centrality of the concepts of environment, host and agent, concepts fundamental to the understanding of health in general. In the above we have given some examples of the ways in which new genetic knowledge and techniques can raise fundamental questions about the nature of these concepts. The new genetics suggests that these relatively stable concepts, which are often seen as fundamentally 'natural' categories, may each be deconstructed or reworked (in theory or practice) or produced. Environment, host and agent may become a part of 'cultivated nature'.

In describing the introduction of newer genetic technologies as part of larger networks, or actor-networks, we are drawing a picture that counters over-simplified genetic reductionist accounts of this new science and technology. Recent conceptions of the environment, and of the body and the subject, have also adopted notions of networks and systems to understand the complexity of construction of concepts such as these. Far from presenting themselves to us in science and other forms of knowing, the environment and the host are produced as the outcome of a web of social relationships. Technologies have the capacity to make such contingent patterns of relationships appear solid, non-contingent, beyond question or natural. Rather like ideologies, these technologies frame a particular view of health and disease. They enforce epistemological assumptions and are contributive to, though *not* determining of, paradigm shifts. The new genetic technologies are capable of 'enframing' our notions of life and of nature in ways that justify new sets of relationships and new forms of governance. The varieties of opposition to biotechnologies illustrate counter-strategies.

It is difficult to see how the 'new genetics' will finally impact upon public health. Currently there would appear to be considerable turbulence in the field and little evidence of stable techno-social networks (Parisi and Terranova, 2000). Rather, there are competing visions of the use of this new technology and knowledge, and there are competing attempts to stabilize the network, in relation to the host, the environment and the agent. By considering the public health field as a sociotechnical network, we are made aware of the broad implications for the field and for society at large. The new genetic technologies in human and non-human genetics draw into question the ways in which we consider the host, agent and environment, and the relationship between these founding concepts. In so doing , they are reconfiguring notions of the social and the demarcation of the public and the private. These developments are occurring within and outside of the public health arena and involve a wide variety of actors.

Chapter 4

The new genetics and the media

Alan Petersen

This chapter focuses on news media portrayals of the new genetics and its applications in the advancement of 'the public's' health. Thus far, there has been relatively little systematic analysis of how the news media help shape public definitions of genetics, and its benefits and risks. This is surprising since the media is a major source of information on genetics and its implications for treatment and prevention, and occupies a crucial position at the interface between scientists and lay publics, serving to translate and disseminate expert knowledge. Indeed, as many sociologists and cultural theorists have argued, in contemporary societies the institutions of the media play a central role in 'mediating' *all* knowledge. As societies have become more complex, communication involving face-to-face encounters has been increasingly replaced by communication involving second-hand reports: firstly, via written forms, such as books, magazines, and newspapers, and then more and more via electronic means, such as fax, television, telephone, and the Internet. For many people, espe-cially in the rich industrialized world, reality has become a 'virtual reality' in that their knowledge of many events and circumstances is gained largely from diverse 'second-hand' sources. However, such 'virtual reality' can have 'real' effects in that it may influence how people think about and act upon issues that profoundly shape their own and others' lives. This is no less the case with genetic knowledge.

The uptake of genetic ideas in preventive medicine and public health is occurring during a period in which there is a burgeoning amount of information on new genetic 'breakthroughs' in the media, linked in particular to various 'gene-mapping' initiatives, such as the HGP. The media constitutes an important element of the cultural context in which new genetic ideas are being taken up and applied in practice. It is likely to influence assessments made of the implications of new 'discoveries', of their benefits and risks, and of the policies or practices that need to be implemented. News media and other media do not just report scientific 'facts'. They convey particular images of science, scientists and nature, and portray possibilities for future actions. They may help raise people's expectations as well as fuel people's fears about the dangers of new genetic technologies. More often than not, news stories of genetic research 'breakthroughs' include some assessment of the implications of research for 'the public's' health and wellbeing. Appeals to the benefits or risks to 'the public' provide a strong motivation for political action and the development of policies. For example, media reports about the cloning of Dolly the sheep, which included claims about the research's implications for human cloning, were met with expressions of outrage and calls by politicians, the Vatican and others to ban research on human cloning, even before the scientific claims had been fully assessed. Debates about the ethics of conducting particular lines of genetic research have, in the past, polarized after the announcement in the press of some new genetic 'breakthrough', without any apparent confirmation of the veracity of the claims, or thorough evaluation of the implications of the research. The news media would appear to play a significant role in setting the agenda of public debate, especially when alternative perspectives are scarce or absent. With the increasing centralization of the institutions of the news media and their agencies, the scope for alternative opinion has narrowed, thereby limiting the opportunities for publics to engage critically with the information with which they are presented. By 'framing' issues as they do – by selectively presenting some issues, themes, facts and claims, while systematically ignoring others – and thereby inviting certain interpretations, the news media are likely to exert powerful effects on their readers or audiences (Priest, 1994: 168). This chapter begins by clarifying our perspective on the media and its portrayal of science and technology in general. It then examines how the media depicts genetic research, and its applications in treatment and prevention in particular, drawing on data derived mainly from a recent study involving major Australian metropolitan newspapers.

The media, science and technology

The term 'the media' is charged with multiple meanings, and this has been the source of some confusion in discussions. Since the

1950s 'the media' has come often to be used in the singular rather than the plural (Williams, 1976: 170), which, for the sake of convenience, will be adhered to in what follows. While in 'popular' usage 'the media' is often viewed as synonymous with the news media, in contemporary communication and cultural studies the media may include a diverse array of communication means or technologies, including books, advertising, the Internet, films, videos, CDs, the telephone, faxes, magazines, professional journals, and pamphlets. Clearly, 'the media' constitutes a rapidly expanding field of communication tools that is less and less constrained by place, time, and particular technologies. The development and rapid diffusion of new means of communication, particularly the Internet and fax, has meant that the dissemination of information to geographically distant locations is instantaneous. There is an increasing convergence of various forms of media, with the result that the distinction between print and electronic media is becoming blurred. Professional journals, for example, are often published simultaneously in 'hard' and electronic versions.

Although the media is increasingly pervasive, it is difficult and hazardous to make generalizations about the impact of the media on 'public opinion' and public policies. For a start, even if one assumes that 'the media' can be clearly defined and delimited, 'it' is always going to be but one factor in a diverse range of factors that contribute to the formation of views and actions. Much discussion about the media, however, has been preoccupied with the question of the media's 'effect' on readers' or audiences' values, attitudes and behaviours, as though the media's influence is certain and profound. Reflecting the liberal humanist assumption that subjects are 'naturally' free and autonomous, albeit constrained by their environments, the media has been consistently identified as a key influence over opinions and actions. Implicit in many discussions is a conception of the subject as a relatively passive, uncritical 'consumer' of information, and a belief that the media 'distorts' some underlying reality. Marxists, for example, have tended to see the media as an agent of propaganda, which serves not only to induce the population to buy the products of capitalist production, but also to obscure the reality of capitalist social relations. The so-called 'media effects' research that has long dominated the academic area of media studies has also tended to assume that media messages and images may serve to 'brainwash' or adversely influence subjects, and so constrain 'freedom of action', one of the taken-for-granted and cherished values of liberal democratic societies. In liberal democracies, the media is seen to play a key role in informing and enlightening citizens about their society, including new scientific and technological developments, unfettered by bias, prejudice, or discrimination. Liberal individualism posits a close connection between the promotion of individual liberty and access to information via a 'free' press; that is, a press independent of the influence of the state or of sectional interests.

Given its perceived role in informing and enlightening citizens, it is hardly surprising that the media in general, and the news media in particular, has been of concern to scholars who study and seek to promote 'the public's' knowledge and comprehension of science and technology. In the research field of 'the public understanding of science', scholars have focused extensively on the role of the media in 'constructing' public knowledge of science and technology, including genetics (see, for example, Durant *et al.*, 1996). For scholars working in this area, the media is seen as playing a potentially key role in shaping public discourse about science and technology, and hence has been identified as a crucial site for analysis of how new knowledge becomes incorporated into the 'common sense' representations of particular social groups. While media coverage of scientific, including genetic, 'breakthroughs' has been pervasive, it would be wrong to assume that the media are all-powerful, and influence views on science and technology in any simple or direct way. For a start, since the media constitutes an increasingly important site for definitional struggles in liberal democratic societies, it is likely to reflect a diverse array of issues, themes and images. Different groups vie for the coverage of issues that they see as best serving their own particular interests. Recognizing this political role of the media, some critical scholars of contemporary media have analysed the media as a site where claims-makers compete to present their own definition of 'the problem' (see Hansen, 2000). There have been a number of recent empirical studies of how different media 'frame' particular problems, for example in the area of environmental politics (e.g. Allan *et al.*, 2000).

The view that the media is all-powerful can be questioned further on the grounds that it assumes that readers or audiences (usually conceived as constituting part of a unitary 'public') are powerless or lacking agency, and that people use and respond to the media in a similar way. Much research on the media undertaken by those interested in the 'public understanding of science', for instance, begins from the premise that people are empty vessels, or passive recipients of information, and are uninformed or ignorant of the expert 'facts'. This 'cognitive deficit' model disregards the extent to which 'life-world' experience shapes people's interest in, and ability to understand, scientific and technical information (Davison *et al.*, 1997: 333). It denies the legitimacy of lay people's ways of reasoning and their non-expert or 'lay knowledge' of science, which may include awareness of its wide-ranging moral, religious, economic, social, and political implications. In a recent UK study of 'lay perspectives' on the new genetics, participants were found to have highly sophisticated views of genetics, health, and risk (Kerr *et al.*, 1998a, 1998b). As in writings on the media more generally, studies on the role of the media in the public understanding of science very frequently posit a direct relationship between the reporting or portrayal of information and the formation of attitudes and behaviours. The assumption that there exists a relatively unitary 'public', with a particular set of characteristics, propensities, and rationalities, denies the range of 'interested publics', groups or associations with interests in science and biotechnology (Davison *et al.*, 1997: 331–2). 'Public understanding is a highly amorphous term, and begs the question of exactly *which* public is being referred to. People differ in terms of their nationality, culture, sex, age, education, occupation and countless other respects, which significantly influence their fund of knowledge, their views and beliefs' (Reiss and Straughan, 1996: 232). Issues of context, including the availability of counter-argument and disconfirming information, and the social backgrounds and particular experiences of readers or audiences, are likely to affect how people interpret and act upon information derived from the media.

Scientists and the media

The relationship between scientists and the media is also more complex than has been portrayed by many writers. According to the dominant 'popularization model' of science communication, transmitting medical news is a one-way information flow beginning with refereed medical journals, expert physicians, and public health officials, who provide medical information to journalists who then popularize specialized biomedical knowledge for lay readers and viewers (Logan, 1991: 44). This suggests that journalists merely interpret and disseminate scientific knowledge to non-scientists. Studies based upon this diffusion model of science popularization generally conclude that not enough information was published, and that what was published was not provided in sufficient quantity or detail to have been useful (Lewenstein, 1995: 347). The implication is that there is a clear boundary between 'science' and 'popularization', which denies the input of popular views into the research process, which affects scientists' beliefs about the content and conduct of science. A point which proponents of the 'popularization' model overlook is that simplification is an intrinsic part of scientific work, both in the laboratory and in communicating with students, funding sources, and specialists in different fields (Hilgartner, 1990: 523–4). The 'popularization' model is underpinned by social learning theory, which denies the influence of social values and scientific decision-making that occurs at every level of biomedical enquiry (Logan, 1991: 56).

As Hilgartner argues, despite conceptual and empirical problems with the dominant view of 'popularization', and consequently its limitations as an analytic tool, it remains a useful political tool for scientific experts (1990: 530). In particular, it has served as a useful rhetorical device for the 'boundary work' (Gieryn, 1983, 1995) of scientists: for demarcating the boundary between 'genuine' (read pure) knowledge and 'popularized' (read contaminated) knowledge, and thus shoring up an idealized view of genuine, objective, scientifically certified knowledge (Hilgartner, 1990: 520). As has been found in the area of the new genetics, scientists are likely to draw such rhetorical boundaries in their efforts to counter what they perceive as unfair press or negative public perceptions of their research (Kerr et al., 1997, 1998c). By setting aside genuine scientific authority as belonging to a realm that cannot be accessed by the public, 'popularization' serves to buttress the epistemic authority of scientists against challenges from outsiders. The flexibility of the boundary between appropriate simplification and distortion allows scientists broad discretion about which aspects of a subject to simplify, how much to simplify, what language and metaphors to use in simplified accounts, and the selection of criteria to be used in matching presentations to their audiences. This discretion allows scientists to present their work in a way that persuades audiences to support their goals (Hilgartner, 1990: 531).

Scientists and science journalists often draw on the rhetoric of popularization when complaining about news media 'distortion' of findings reported in scientific journals. As scientists and science journalists are frequently at pains to point out, professional journals publish articles that are the product of a process of rigorous 'peer-review', with articles published only after a lengthy process, sometimes involving further research, revision, and reappraisal. This is seen to ensure the objectivity and validity of the data. The news media, on the other hand, are seen to place a premium on the 'scoop' or 'exclusive', and publish articles under tight constraints of time, space, and the need to simplify complex information. This is considered to introduce an element of subjectivity that is likely to lead to 'distortion' of 'the facts'. For example, in a recent editorial the deputy editor of *The New England Journal of Medicine* emphasized differences between journals and the news media in their aims and modus operandi, pointing out how this is likely to affect news reporting. The deputy editor was responding to a study of newspaper and television coverage of three medications used to prevent major diseases, which showed numerous instances in which stories contained inadequate or incomplete information about the benefits, risks, and costs associated with the medications (Steinbrook, 2000: 1669). As the deputy editor notes:

Only a minority of the articles we [NEJM] publish each year are widely publicized outside the medical community. Although we are pleased when our articles receive wide attention, we do not select them to make headlines. Nevertheless, if we do our job as editors well, a newspaper, magazine, or television report on a journal article is likely to be more reliable than it would have been had the article not gone through the peer-review and revision process.... Journalists need to translate detailed and complicated medical papers into succinct stories that are easy to understand, yet they must provide context and balance and omit nothing that is really important. This can be very difficult. Many articles are written against a deadline, and a comprehensive article may have to be written in an hour or two. Editors sometimes shorten reports about medicine, and important information may be omitted. A reader has no way of knowing whether the reporter failed to include the relevant information or an editor cut it out.

(Steinbrook, 2000: 1669)

Despite their frequent criticisms of news media for their reporting of science 'fact', scientists are acutely aware of their reliance on the media and the need to maintain a good relationship with journalists. Genetic researchers in particular are keen to use the media to promote the importance of their work and to improve their public image in order to assure continuity of public funding for their research and to counter negative images of genetics shaped by its historical association with eugenics (Nelkin, 1994: 25–6). In their effort to counter public scepticism about genetics and its bene-fits, and to enhance their prestige and competitive advantage in new fields of research, scientists have sought to gain greater control over science news and the images that they present. To this end, they have made increasing use of public relations experts to promote favourable images of genetics (Nelkin, 1985). In the US at least, a journal such as *Nature* seeks to obtain maximum attention for its articles by having virtually every newspaper and television show in the country reporting on one or more of its articles on the very day the journal is published (Kolata, 1997: 26). In order to give reporters a head start on their articles, journals send out informa-tion to journalists about articles in forthcoming issues several days in advance of publication. This may be by way of press releases, abstracts, or early copies of the forthcoming issue. This information is generally embargoed until the date of publication (Steinbrook, 2000: 1669). Sometimes the release of information might be delayed because of a confidentiality agreement with a sponsoring commer-cial organization, or a pending patent application, as was the case with the announcement of the cloning of the sheep Dolly (see Kolata, 1997: 26–30).

Scientists seek to gain control over the portrayal of their research by employing particular metaphors that both help convey complex ideas to a broad lay public and communicate the excitement and the benefits of their work (Nelkin, 1994: 25–6; Van Dijck, 1998: 11–12). As Van Dijck explains, the choice of metaphors is always strategic, and scientists as well as journalists have always been keenly aware of the impact of metaphors on the public's understanding of science (1998: 23). Many scientists are employed by the biotechnology industry, which has actively sought to convey positive images of genetics through the mass media in order to boost public expectations about treatments and investors' expectations of profits (Hubbard and Wald, 1997: 2; Van Dijck, 1998: 104–10). Although genetic researchers, and the professional journals in which they publish, seek to promote a view of research as objective, value-free, and rigorous, scientific descriptions rely heavily on imagery and metaphors circulating in the broader culture, and reflect social biases and assumptions. Articles appearing in mass-circulation science journals such as *Nature*, *Science*, *New Scientist*, *Scientific American*, and *Science News*, which provide the source for many stories on genetics in the mainstream news media, have been found to draw extensively on popular imagery and metaphors, and to contain gender and heterosexist biases (Petersen, 1999).

Journalists, on the other hand, despite claims to being independent, are often under personal and institutional pressures to conform to scientific values. Their scientific writing is thus likely to reflect the concerns of the scientific community rather than the concerns of the 'public', whom they frequently profess to represent. The popular science produced by science journalists is likely to reinforce a vision of science as a coherent body of knowledge about an underlying objective reality – an image that is at odds with contemporary ideas about the social construction of scientific knowledge (Lewenstein, 1995: 345). Journalists need to maintain a good relationship with scientists, on whom they rely to identify and validate stories. Because they are under intense deadline pressures, journalists need the protection offered by appeals to scientific objectivity. They seldom have the time, confidence, or expertise to independently verify 'the truth', and hence rely on an appearance of impartiality to fend off criticism (Miller and Riechert, 2000: 50). Some journalists do not have the skills to critically evaluate scientific research (Logan, 1991: 47). Consequently, they are compelled to take some information on trust and to rely on technical sources of information (Nelkin, 1987: 86; Karpf, 1988: 125).

The press, like its readers, generally finds science intimidating, so editors are likely to insist on the sources that have obvious credentials and credibility (Goodell, 1986: 177). Journalists tend to rely on established, pre-packaged sources for news within governments, large health facilities, well-established medical journals, and large research universities, and on staged events that are often managed by public relations offices within hospitals, clinics, journals or physicians' interest groups (Logan, 1991: 47). The reliance on well-established experts, combined with the emphasis on staged events, results in the neglect of the sociological, cultural, ethical, historical and educational contexts underlying medical news (Logan, 1991: 48). In a British study of science and medical journalists in the British national press, it was found that journalists apply a register of explicit and implicit criteria in the process of determining the credibility of individual scientists and their claims (Hansen, 1994). This ranges from explicit criteria, such as rank, qualifications, publications record, and institution, to more subjective criteria, such as 'gut feeling' about the research or the scientist, or 'what kinds of personalities they are' (Hansen, 1994: 122–3). The one type of reporting that was found to depart from this normal routine of assessing credibility and validity is the reporting of research published in peer-reviewed scientific journals. As Hansen argues, this is one area where science journalism seems to differ markedly from other kinds of journalism. As Hansen notes: 'If coverage is based on an article published in peer-reviewed scientific journals, the journalists do not see any need for checking – and often articles would be written without contacting the authors for other than "colourful" or "good" quotes, and certainly without cross-checking with other scientists' (1994: 123).

As should be evident from the above, the 'mediation' of scientific knowledge involves a complex series of 'behind-the-scenes' negotiations between scientists and journalists. The outcome of these negotiations will affect what gets covered in 'the news' and also to some extent how stories are portrayed, since the use of particular language and of accompanying illustrative material is also subject to negotiation. Journalists' and scientists' views on the perceived 'newsworthiness' of stories clearly constitute an important factor among a diverse array of factors that are likely to affect what aspects of research get reported and how they are reported. In recent years the findings of genetic research have become highly 'newsworthy' because they are seen by both scientists and news editors to be of wide interest to 'the public'. The area of health and medicine in general is seen to be of intrinsic interest, especially in light of the vast amount of public expenditure in this area (Karpf, 1988). However, genetic research in particular is seen as being of great interest, since it is seen as contributing to the next revolution or 'new wave' in treatment and prevention. Because of the perceived potential of genetics in preventive intervention, prenatal health, and the curing of a range of acute and chronic diseases, genetic research appears to directly address enduring concerns such as the health of offspring, the effects of ageing, and the burgeoning costs of medical treatment. Rarely a day goes by without the announcement of some new gene discovery or of a likely new genetic-based treatment or prevention strategy. The claim is sometimes of a general nature, such as a promised revolution or 'golden era' in treatments or prevention per se, often announced in the titles of articles:

'Biotechnology enters golden era' (Tanner, 1999)
'Biotechnology is the next great wave' (Meredith, 2000)

More often the focus is placed on a particular area of research that has a likely 'spin-off' for the treatment or prevention of a particular condition:

'Gene discovery may alleviate obesity, diabetes' (Brook, 2001)
'New gene joins cancer battle' (*The Weekend Australian*, 29–30
    January 2000: 7)
'Gene therapy for heart vessels' (Hickman, 1999)
'Scientists hail gene therapy that fights cancer tumours' (Meek,
    2000)
'Scientists head for a genetic disorder pill' (*The West Australian*, 3
    October 1998: 40)

The prominence of gene stories

In a study of newspaper portrayals of genetics and medicine in three Australian newspapers – *The Australian*, *The Sydney Morning Herald (SMH)*, and *The West Australian (The West)* – in the late 1990s, gene stories were found to be prominent (see Petersen, 2001). This study, which covers a period in which a number of widely publicized genetic 'breakthroughs' were announced, including the cloning of Dolly (in February 1997) and numerous discoveries arising from the Human Genome Project and similar 'gene-mapping' initiatives, provides the bulk of the data for the discussion which follows. Although the study found that gene stories appeared only occasionally in the headlines on the first page, a large proportion of articles appear in the first three pages, while the majority of articles appeared in the first ten pages. The prominence of gene stories in each of the newspapers highlights that editors see these stories as highly newsworthy. Gene stories often appear in special feature sections of the newspapers, particularly those focusing on health and medical issues. In *The Australian* many articles are published in sections focusing on health, technology, and national and international affairs, particularly in the weekend edition (*The Weekend Australian*), where detailed reports often feature in 'The Medical Review'. Stories appearing in this section are likely to appeal to readers with a more specialist interest in health and medical issues. In the case of the *SMH* and *The West,* articles are much less likely to appear in special feature sections of the newspaper; however, articles on genetic research can often be seen alongside other articles dealing with health or medical issues, thereby constituting a de facto health and medical section. For example, in one edition of the *SMH* a series of articles as found under the heading 'The cost of living: science tackles the problem of ageing in the hope of curbing health costs' (*SMH*, 31 March 1998: 1, 4).

Many articles cite or quote scientists, who explain the nature and significance of the research and/or its findings and its implications for treatment or prevention. These citations or quotes lend credibility to stories by conveying the impression that the information is unmediated – straight from the expert's mouth – and hence irrefutable. The source of the citation or quote is usually someone of authority, such as a scientist or a director from a prestigious institute. Peter Conrad, who has interviewed science and medicine reporters in the US about their use of expert sources, argues that journalists select quotes to support a perspective, to say things that they can't say, for example that a piece of research has limited importance, or is likely to have particular outcomes. As he observes, quotes operate as journalistic tools that are likely to influence readers' perceptions of reality and perceptions of issues (Conrad, 1999: 292–3, 300). They are often detailed accounts of the nature and significance of the research, as in the following excerpt from a story about a clinical trial (described as 'a radical new treatment') involving a gene therapy for sufferers of mesothelioma.

> Director of research at the hospital, Professor Bruce Robinson, said the injections stimulated the production of the cytokine gene, which in turn activated 'killer cells' to eliminate the cancer. 'The rationale is you get maximum effect in the tumour, minimum side effects and it's much better for the patient because they don't have to hang around in hospital,' he said.

Professor Robinson said there was a 'reasonable' chance the therapy, a world-first in mesothelioma treatment, would be successful. If so, he said, it could be used to treat other 'solid' cancers, including breast cancer. 'Gene therapy is what you might call the cutting edge of modern cancer developments,' he said. '(But) it's a bit like prospecting – you know there's gold down there, but you don't know which hole you dig is going to find it'.

(Green, 1996: 7)

This article, like many others, relies heavily on the scientist's own descriptions and (positive) evaluations, and provides no independent confirmation of the research or its significance. Since no alternative perspective is presented, there is little reason for the reader to doubt the veracity of the scientist's claims. In articles where other scientists' views are presented, these tend to confirm or elaborate on, rather than challenge, what has been said. The generally positive portrayal of genetic research is undoubtedly due, in part, to the aforementioned fact that journalists rely heavily on single, pre-packaged sources for news and on staged events where scientists and public relations people control the flow of information. Articles sometimes indicate that the news source was a special event such as a scientific conference, the launch of a new genetics research unit, or the release of a discussion paper. These events provide the context and opportunity for researchers to announce or discuss the findings of new genetics research and their significance. The lack of independent confirmation and critical commentary can also be partly explained by the fact that journalists very often rely on information published in peer-reviewed scientific journals for their stories. Journals such as *New Scientist, Nature, Science, Nature Genetics, The Lancet, The New England Journal of Medicine, Immunity,* and *Nature Medicine* are cited as sources in many of the articles. Journalists see publications such as these as highly credible sources that do not require independent verification (Hansen, 1994: 123).

Stories of discovery

Discoveries are part-and-parcel of the scientific endeavour, and so it should be of no surprise that a significant number of articles in each of the newspapers report the discovery of a new gene, a gene link, a gene mutation, or the 'functions' of a gene. These discovery stories are very often written by regular medical or science writers, and would seem to follow a fairly standard pattern of reporting. In many instances these stories announce clearly in bold titles that there has been a discovery, for example through the use of phrases such as 'gene find/ing', 'gene identified', 'gene/s link/ed', 'genetic link/s', or 'discovery of gene':

'Gene find may lead to vaccine for malaria' (Hawkes, 1996)
'Cancer gene identified' (Hickman, 1998a)
'New genes linked with cancer cells' (Hickman, 1998b)
'Genetic link to disease' (Hickman, 1998c)
'Discovery of mutant gene offers HIV hope' (Larriera, 1996)
'Discovery of bowel cancer gene gives hope of prevention' (Dayton, 1997a)
'Genetic links spark hope for obese' (*SMH*, 24 June, 1997: 3)

On other occasions, however, titles only vaguely allude to a new gene 'discovery', and readers need to read past the titles, and sometimes well into the article, to learn of the nature of the discovery.

The frequent use of words such as 'found', 'discovered', 'located', 'identified', 'isolated' and 'pinpointed' in news reports leaves little doubt about the existence of a gene and/or its location. For example, one article ('Gene find brings hope for glaucoma sufferers') begins with the comment that 'Australian and American doctors have *identified a gene* responsible for the eye disorder glaucoma...', and then goes on to say that researchers 'have *pinpointed the gene* that blocks the removal of fluid from the eye, causing a severe form of glaucoma' (Harris, 1997: 52; emphases added). An article reporting research on a virus that killed a United States Army private during the Spanish flu outbreak of 1918–19 ('Long-dead soldier gives clue to deadliest epidemic') notes that the US Army team (of scientists) 'nailed the killer by *isolating five of its genes*' (Dayton, 1997b: 8; emphases added). These descriptions reinforce the perception that our health problems originate inside us and draw attention away from external factors that need to be addressed (Hubbard and Wald, 1997: 5). They are based on the reductionist assumption that the smallest things can have the most overwhelming effects (1997: 3). In some articles the identified gene is clearly ascribed a causative role; that is, the gene is described as being 'responsible' for or as 'causing' a disease, or as 'protecting' people from disease. However, at other times a causative role is simply implied, as when the gene is described as being 'implicated in developing' a disease or as being 'linked to' a disease.

Unlocking nature's secrets

Geneticists are frequently portrayed, and when quoted often portray themselves, as being involved in a quest to unlock nature's secrets. The use of words such as 'secrets' and 'mysteries' in descriptions of genetic research, by suggesting that the scientific process has an incommunicable or esoteric quality, serves rhetorically to buttress the authority and mystique of science. In his article 'The dawning of a new age of therapy', the scientist Sir Gustav Nossal states that: 'Problems that had previously seemed entirely impenetrable, such as birth defects, genetic diseases, cancer and aging, are *yielding up their biochemical and cellular secrets*' (Nossal, 1998: 4; emphases added). In another article, 'Prognosis of a whole country', it is announced that: 'One of the remotest corners of Europe is *poised to reveal the Holy Grail of medical research: the genetic cause of disease*'. (The article reports that Iceland was to 'give a private research company exclusive access to every citizen's health records' as part of research into the genetic basis of disease.) The article then goes on to say: 'The data, cross-referenced with DNA samples and genealogical records going back to the sagas, *could reveal the fundamental mysteries of existence*.' (Binyon, 1999: 39; emphases added). These descriptions ascribe researchers with divine qualities; they hold secrets known only to the initiated and are capable of performing miracles. The reference to the 'Holy Grail' above is a recurring element in popular stories on the Human Genome Project, and presents an image of scientific research as a quest for a mysterious treasure (Van Dijck, 1998: 21, 128).

The use of metaphors such as 'puzzle', 'riddle', 'code', 'book' or 'map' in descriptions of the human genome, and of terms such as 'decoding', 'code-breaking' and 'map-making' in accounts of genetic research, are widespread in news stories, as they are in 'popular' (i.e. mass-circulation) science journal articles (Petersen, 1999). It is likely that these metaphors are imported directly from these journals, which, as mentioned, are often the cited sources for stories, or from the scientists who are interviewed. The use of these metaphors in descriptions lends credence to the view that scientific research is an objective search for an underlying reality; an incremental uncovering of the facts. This can be seen clearly in an article focusing on recent research developments in genetics, 'Genetic jigsaw falls neatly into place' (Amalfi, 1999a: 17). In the article it is noted that: 'The first working draft [of the complete book of human genes] should be available by February with the *last pieces of the genetic jigsaw* expected to be completed by 2003' (emphases added). Another article ('Gene genie') notes that the Human Genome Project will have 'far reaching implications, perhaps leading to gene therapies for many diseases' and 'could also provide *answers to the riddles* of ageing and death' (Callaghan, 1996: 2; emphases added).

It is not always easy to tell who originally introduced a particular analogy or metaphor – whether it was the scientist who is cited or quoted, or the journalist who wrote the story. In some articles, however, it would appear that the scientist originally used the analogy or metaphor, which was then adopted or modified by the journalist. This is evident, for example, in a news article announcing that a scientist (described as a 'genetic map-maker') 'has perfected a 'colour-coded "street guide" that promises to detect cellular hotspots likely to cause cancers and other abnormalities'. Here there is a mixing of the metaphors of the 'code' and of the 'map' that appear in the scientist's own description. In the article the scientist is cited as saying that 'the new screening technique comple-mented black and white strips of DNA *resembling bar codes used on shopping centre goods*'. He is also quoted as saying: '*Without the maps you do not know where to go....* They have immediate applica-tions in clinical work, where *the coloured bar codes* can identify changes or rearrangements in the chromosomes.' (*The West*, 25 July 1997: 10; emphases added). The scientists who are frequently quoted in the articles, or who are authors of articles, make liberal use of such metaphors in their efforts to help the reader conceptu-alize that which is as yet non-existent, that is, too abstract, too tiny, or too large to describe in ordinary language. By transferring everyday language into a complex scientific concept, they at least give lay readers the illusion that they understand the basic mecha-nism of genetics or the process of research (Van Dijck, 1998: 22).

The significance of metaphors in helping readers both visualize complex, molecular-level processes and appreciate the complexity and significance of genetic research is particularly explicit in the following description of the Human Genome Project ('Genetic code-breakers'), written by the co-authors/scientists Craig Venter and Daniel Cohen:

> For the first time, we will have a complete description of life at the most fundamental level of the genetic code. This map will describe for us the exact content and structure, not only of each and every gene associated with a species, but also the precoded information, or 'chemical spelling', that controls when a particular gene is turned 'on' or 'off', leading to a biological effect.... The human genome is 1.5 m long and has 3 billion letters, all of which are likely to be decoded, along with the genomes of hundreds of other species, by 2005. The millions to billions of letters in the genetic code of each species, from ourselves to the simplest bacteria, contain the recorded history of 4.2 billion years of evolution. With every gene identified and every letter of the chemical spelling deciphered, we will be able to see the exact differences at the genetic level – not just the physical level observed by Darwin and evolutionary scientists to this day – between any two species. How humans are different from other species, and how they are not, will finally be revealed.
>
> (Venter and Cohen, 1997: 28)

Here a number of metaphors and analogies are used to assist the authors in communicating complex scientific information. The use of the metaphors of the 'code' and the 'map', and of the words 'letters' and 'chemical spelling', provides a ready-made imagery for readers who are assumed unlikely to have either the vocabulary or the expertise to grasp easily the complexity of the genetic 'deciphering' or 'decoding' task. The complexity and momentous significance of genetic research are underlined by phrases such as 'the millions to billions of letters' and 'the recorded history of 4.2 billion years of evolution' – figures that are assumed beyond the imagination of lay people. However geneticists – the 'code breakers' – are seen to have acquired techniques of visualization that allow 'a complete description of life at the most fundamental level of the genetic code'. Thus, unlike 'Darwin and other evolutionary scientists to this day', whose powers of visualization were restricted to 'the physical level', geneticists 'will be able to see the exact differences at the genetic level ... between any two species'.

In this description the metaphorical and literal have become blurred, so that it is difficult to recognize the ways in which the metaphors invite certain interpretations and not others. As Van Dijck observes, the use of the metaphors of the 'map' and the 'code' has become so ingrained in genetics that they have begun to lose their figurative meaning, and to serve as literal terms (1998: 22). The apparent precision of the map and of the code make invisible the priorities and interests that have shaped them. The map imagery suggests that once a gene is located, its interpretation will be objective and independent of context:

> A mapped gene may appear to be a straightforward detail, to be extracted and understood without reference to culture and experience. Yet the language of the genome, like the language of the dictionary, must be contextualised to be understood. Genes are, like words, products of (evolutionary) history, dependent on context, and often ambiguous, open to more than one interpretation.
>
> (Nelkin and Lindee, 1995: 9)

Neglect of non-genetic and 'multifactorial' explanations

Rarely do news reports mention the influence of non-genetic factors and 'multifactorial' interactions on disorders. Despite the recognition by many molecular geneticists that diseases are 'multifactorial' and have an experiential or environmental component (Limoges, 1994: 121–2), only a few articles on genetic research acknowledge this. In discussions where environmental influences are mentioned, references tend to be made only in passing and, in most cases, well into the article or towards the end of the article. In one report ('Genetics hold key to beating cancer') an expert states that '90 percent of cancers were caused by genes damaged after birth through environmental influences' (Ferrari, 1997: 51), while in another ('Childless may demand cloning') an expert comments that: 'If it [cloning] did occur, the cloned individuals would not be "clones" in the sense of being completely identical', since the 'mother's influence, brain development and other random events such as early sensory experience would still determine personal development' (Debelle, 1998: 5). In neither article is there discussion about the implications of these non-genetic influences for further research, or treatment or prevention. A third article, which announces that 'Australian researchers hope to develop a test for migraine after identifying two genes causing it' ('Genes clue to relief'), acknowledges that the 'underlying cause for migraine is genetic, but common triggers include red wine, ripe cheese and chocolate' (Chynoweth, 1998). Again there is no discussion of the relative contribution of these 'non-genetic' ('life-style') influences, and of the implications for prevention or treatment.

Furthermore, there is never mention of the fact that the disorder may be the product of the *interaction* of a number of genes. Although many scientists subscribe to the notion that diseases are likely to be the outcome of interaction among several or many genes, as well as between those genes and the surrounding biological context (see, for example, Cranor, 1994: 133), stories fail to convey a sense of this dynamic and complexity. As Cranor (1994) argues, because causal explanations are so context- and interest-dependent, it is important to scrutinize causal ascriptions carefully for their contexts and for the aims such ascriptions might serve. Such causal notions are frequently invoked to make a normative point, instead of arguing for the research or the therapeutic point more directly. Thus, as Cranor suggests, scientists may, in some cases, emphasize genetic causation as part of a deliberate persuasive strategy; as a tool to convince people to focus on certain therapies (1994: 129, 136).

Good news stories

Many gene discoveries would seem to make the news, and be given prominence, precisely because they are good news stories; that is, they are seen to offer solutions to health problems. Such stories, conveying genetic optimism, have been found to dominate news coverage of genetics and mental illness in the US from the mid-1980s, and to persist even where the most promising claims could not be replicated or were subsequently retracted (Conrad, 2001). The prominence given such stories is assisted, no doubt, by scientists themselves, who, as mentioned, are keen to promote the benefits of genetics research in order to ensure ongoing funding for research and to alleviate public concerns about the outcomes of research. Genetic research is very frequently portrayed as offering hope for new treatments, tests, or (less often) preventive strategies. On the other hand, potential disadvantages and dangers are either ignored or provide only a minor sub-theme. As in media depictions of health and medicine more generally, news reports on genetic research contain many stories of breakthroughs and triumphs that suggest that today's diseases will be vanquished tomorrow (Karpf, 1988: 139). Articles make frequent reference to scientists' predictions of new diagnostic tests, new drugs or vaccines, or new genetic therapies resulting from research, often including their predictions about the likely time of their availability. An article on Alzheimer's disease ('Potential exists for early Alzheimer's cure') predicts that: 'Early-onset Alzheimer's would become a preventable disorder with potential cures being tested within five years.' It goes on to report that a US research team had developed a genetic test for Alzheimer's which promised to be '100 per cent accurate' (McGuirk, 1997: 50). Another article, on Friedreich's Ataxia, 'a degenerative neurological disease that results in total loss of body coordination', cites a medical geneticist who 'says it is likely treatment could become available in the next 10 years following the discovery of the causal gene by a group of doctors from France, America, Italy and Canada' (Reiner, 1999: 17).

The newsworthiness of a story is considerably enhanced if it is linked to an issue that has already been established as being of major public concern, such as the crisis in health care funding. Hence the prominence given to a series of articles appearing in an edition of the *SMH* which explores the potential of genetics to curb health care costs associated with an ageing population (Hill and Dayton, 1998: 1). As is noted in the opening paragraph of the lead story: 'By the time the first baby boomer turns 60, some of the nastiest diseases – including dementia, cancer, cardiovascular conditions, depression, diabetes and osteoporosis – will have revealed their genetic roots.' This is described as having implications not only for accelerating the development of treatments, but also for reducing health care costs, which are predicted to increase with an ageing population. As in other articles, the link between more knowledge about the genetic basis of disease and new or improved treatment is not challenged. Thus, one expert is quoted as saying that: 'Once those genes have been found and their functions worked out ... then it is highly likely that there will be ways of getting around that susceptibility or delaying its effects.' In another article it is noted that: 'More knowledge of disease will lead to more effective technology and drugs, and will tell us more about the progression and complications of disease in the individual' (Hill and Dayton, 1998: 4).

Sometimes the development of treatments is portrayed as imminent. For example, a report ('Revolution in the wings for pre-natal testing') on the development of a new prenatal blood test for genetic disorders, 'PreScreen', notes that 'PreScreen could be on the market as early as next year' (Eccleston, 1998: 3). Another, which announces the discovery of the gene for Parkinson's disease, quotes an Australian scientist as saying that 'he hoped to have a diagnostic test available "within weeks" at the hospital' (Dayton, 1998: 5). The time-line for the development of a treatment is not always precisely defined. For example, an article which announces the identification of 'five genes responsible' for 'the most devastating – and most common – degenerative brain disorders' (neuronal ceroid lipofusci-noses) notes that '*it is only a matter of time* before genetic therapies will be developed by research teams' (Bower, 1997: 54; emphases added). However, doubt is rarely expressed about whether a treatment will eventually be found.

Such stories help lend credence to the belief that experts become more expert, and will find technological solutions for even the most intractable medical problems. They deny uncertainty and death, and bolster expertise, 'suggesting that everything is knowable and conquerable' (Karpf, 1988: 139–40). In many reports geneticists are portrayed as warriors or heroes, as constituting the vanguard of the 'genetics revolution', and as waging a war against disease or 'rogue genes'. An image of the geneticist-as-warrior is strongly evoked in the opening paragraphs of a report, 'Vaccine warrior', which focuses in some detail on the contribution of a geneticist to the development of a DNA vaccine:

> Jeff Boyle has the brave new word of genetics and DNA vaccines at his feet. That much was apparent when in March he had an article published in international science journal *Nature*. For research scientists, publication of their findings in *Nature* is the pinnacle of achievement. Only the best scale it. … In the precise clinical language of learned journals, the headline [of the article] disguises the enormous potential of DNA vaccine research for human health. Hidden in those few words is the contribution of Boyle, Lew and Brady [his colleagues] to the development of a whole new generation of vaccines…. It is timely research. Just as the medical world is crying out for a fresh set of vaccines, along comes a genera-tion of researchers bringing the world another generation of drugs.
>
> (Leech, 1998a: 10)

Images such as this are greatly assisted through the use of military analogies, whereby the scientist is pitted against an evil enemy (a 'killer disease') seen to threaten the public's health. In the above story the vaccine is presented as a weapon that the geneticist-warrior has developed just in time. Consistent with the military analogy, themes of attack, defeat, and capture figure prominently in such descriptions. For example, an article called 'Resistance to drugs cracks' announces that: 'Genetic scientists *are on the verge of defeating life-threatening organisms* that have developed strong resistance to conventional antibiotics, says one of this year's Australia Prize winners' (Leech, 1998b: 40; emphases added). Another article, 'Discovery of bowel cancer gene gives hope of prevention', reports a scientist as saying that another scientist '*may have the human gene in months*' (Ewing, 1997: 6; emphases added).

Military metaphors help convey the importance of the research for the development of new preventive techniques, drugs or therapies. This can be seen in the following report, which comments on the potential of a 'new weapon' to have application in a pre-emptive attack:

> A family of genetically-modified insects is being developed in an attempt to *rid the world of killer diseases*. A designer bug that can no longer pass on Chugs disease, which affects up to 20 million people a year, has been created by scientists who want to use the same technique to *stamp out malaria and dengue fever....* By inserting a gene from another insect that *triggers an attack on the parasite*, biologists are able to get the host insect to react to the parasites it is carrying and *destroy them before they can be passed on to humans*.
>
> (Dobson, 1999: 16; emphases added)

In this news article, and many others, researchers appear as altruistic defenders of the public's health. This image is common in contemporary popular representations of geneticists, as Van Dijck (1998) observes. That is, rather than being seen as 'the wizardy lab worker or the savvy scientist-entrepreneur', the prevalent image is that of 'a doctor in a white coat' who is on a mission to save the lives of innocent victims of congenital disease (1998: 131–2). The use of anthropomorphic terms such as 'rogue genes' and 'killer diseases', which attribute malevolent intent to genes and diseases, reinforces the heroic image of genetic researchers, and bolsters their status as guardians of the public's health. There are few references to the potential dangers posed to health by particular research projects. Although concerns about the ethical implications of genetic research in general, and cloning research in particular, are frequently expressed in articles (see below), the validity of specific research projects is never questioned.

There is little debate about the value of particular lines of genetic research, about whether research can deliver what is promised, and whether funds used for research would be better spent in other ways. Furthermore, few articles make reference to, or comment (critically or otherwise) on, the content of earlier news reports, or refute earlier reported findings. In line with findings of research into the US news media (see Conrad, 1997: 145, 1999: 11–15), the present study found limited reporting of disconfirming evidence in any of the newspapers. That is, the articles provide no sense of dynamism and continuity in the research process, or of ongoing debate about the significance of findings. In all the newspapers there is a strong bias in favour of the positive outcomes of genetic research, and an apparent disinclination to report negative or inconclusive findings. However, despite the generally positive portrayals of genetics and geneticists, it would be wrong to leave the impression that there is no recognition or expression of uncertainty and fear about the consequences of 'tampering with nature'. Underlying concerns about the unintended or unforeseen consequences of genetic research are mirrored in a number of reports, most evidently in those focusing on cloning research.

The portrayal of cloning research: the aftermath of Dolly

Public concerns about scientists 'going too far' were widespread in the aftermath of the announcement of the cloning of the sheep Dolly, in February 1997, and subsequent media reports, in January 1998, that a US scientist, Richard Seed, intended to clone human beings. The extent of media and public interest in Dolly would seem to have few parallels in the history of biotechnology 'breakthroughs'. As Turney notes, the birth of Dolly was viewed as the realization of an idea that had been discussed for more than half a century, although her advent was treated as a great surprise (1998: 214). For example, both the director of the US National Human Genome Research Institute and the president of the US National

Academy of Sciences were reported to have been 'totally caught off guard' by the announcement (Butler and Wadman, 1997: 9). However, what was novel about Dolly, commentators pointed out, was the use of cells that were not embryonic but adult, i.e. 'differentiated' (Nash, 1997: 63). This suggested the possibility of 'turning back the biological clock', or working against the 'laws of nature' – a feat that was, until then, seen as limited to the realms of science fiction. The prospect that the same technique could be applied to humans was viewed as having immense potential – both for medical treatment and for expanding personal life options. By presenting people with the possibility of reproducing themselves, cloning promised immortality and the ability to reproduce oneself asexually – evidently an attractive proposition to the vain, the infertile and many gay and lesbian people who wanted to have children. Dr Ian Wilmut, the leader of the research team that cloned Dolly, was reported as claiming, soon after the announcement of Dolly, that 'hundreds of people, mainly women, have approached him about cloning themselves' (*The Australian*, 4 March 1997: 6). A crucial point that appears to have been overlooked by journalists is the qualification provided by the scientists who cloned Dolly, in their original article, that it was possible that only a small proportion of the differentiated cells would have effective embryonic potential (Gould, 1998: 45–6). From the perspective of the media, this qualification may have been regarded as dampening the impact of an event that was seen by journalists as extremely newsworthy (see Kolata, 1997: 21–35). With the birth of Dolly the sheep 'science fact' was seen to be moving closer to popular images. In its December 1997 editorial, the journal *Science* proclaimed that the cloning of Dolly was one of the major scientific 'breakthroughs' of 1997. That is, it made obsolete 'preconceived limits' in the field of biotechnology and would 'profoundly change the practice or interpretation of science or its implications for society' (Bloom, 1997: 2029).

From very early on in the news coverage, the implications of the research for the cloning of humans, as well as for medicine and agriculture, were drawn, even though details of the research had yet to be published in *Nature*. (The story was broken by a science editor of the *Observer*, who obtained information from a source other than *Nature*, thus technically avoiding breaking the embargo that was in place until the expected date of publication, which was 27 February (Kolata, 1997: 30; Wilmut *et al.*, 2000: 244).) In the article Wilmut himself never spelt out the human cloning implications of the research, nor did the accompanying editorial. The title of Wilmut's article certainly said nothing about clones; it was called 'Viable offspring derived from foetal and adult mammalian cells' (Kolata, 1997: 27). Journalists, however, were quick to draw implications from the research. An article appearing in *The Australian* ('Scientists create first clone of adult animal') noted that: 'The success of the work [the cloning of Dolly] *brings the possibility of human cloning, which is illegal under present laws governing research, one step closer*' (*The Australian*, 24 February 1997: 7; emphases added). In an *SMH* news report, an Australian senior research scientist is quoted: 'If it can be done with sheep *there is every likelihood it can also be done with humans* – entering the Brave New World era in terms of possible uses it can be put to' (Hoy, 1997: 8; emphases added). Alongside this article there appears a short 'Analysis' piece by a journalist who writes that 'whenever previous animal cloning advances have been made *the fearsome prospect of human cloning has been raised*, and rightly so: the ghosts of Hitler and eugenics trigger ghastly memories' (emphases added). In response to the question 'So can we clone humans now?', he responds: 'Technically, who knows? Nature does it often with identical twins' (Beale, 1997: 8; emphases added). In *The West* it was reported that President Clinton 'asked the national ethics board to review the "troubling" implications of the cloning of adult sheep – *a biological feat that might allow the mass production of identical people*' (*The West Australian*, 26 February 1997; emphases added). The article acknowledged that: 'Proponents said the new technology could lead to the creation of farm animals that made human medicines in their milk or contained organs suitable for transplanting into people'; and then went on to say that: 'At its worst, *it could be used by people to create copies of themselves or to make armies of genetically identical slaves*' (*The West Australian*, 26 February 1997; emphases added).

None of these initial articles spelled out in detail the nature of the threat(s) posed by human cloning. However, the use of terms and phrases such as 'Brave New World', 'the ghosts of Hitler and eugenics', 'Master race', 'the production of clones on an industrial scale', 'mass production of identical people', and 'make armies of genetically identical slaves' evokes strong images of social engineering and authoritarian control. Neither in these reports about Dolly, nor in subsequent articles about cloning, was there discussion of the differences between 'popular' meanings of the term 'clone' (i.e. duplication, or cheap imitation of a complete original), and its more specific biological meaning (Silver, 1998: 105–6). Rather, stories and any accompanying visual material, including diagrams of 'how Dolly was developed' and drawings depicting duplication or mirror images, tend to reflect and reinforce the popular image of cloning as duplication or 'imitation'. This can be clearly seen, for example, in the article 'Super-milk cow looms amid fear over tampering', which appeared in *The West* a week after Dolly. The report, which makes reference to the German news magazine *Der Spiegel*, which included a drawing showing five identical copies of Adolf Hitler marching next to four Albert Einsteins, and three Claudia Schiffers, is overshadowed by a large reproduction of the drawing. The validity of the Dolly experiment, or the claims of the scientific team, seemed not to have been independently verified by any of the journalists, even though, as one journalist remarked, the findings were, at the time of the original reports, 'still unpublished, so details are scarce' (Beale, 1997: 8). Although one scientist was reported, in the initial *SMH* article on Dolly, as calling for verification of the findings (Hoy, 1997: 8), none of the articles contain independent confirmatory information, or contending scientific views. The fact that the article was known to have been accepted for publication by a prestigious scientific journal, *Nature*, is likely to have lent legitimacy to the research, which was seen as not requiring verification.

Drawing the line

In the weeks and months following the initial reports, the newspapers were filled with stories about various official responses to the prospects of human cloning. Prominent scientists and authorities were quick to distance themselves from the application of the new technology in human cloning, which was described variously as 'repugnant', 'against nature', and 'against God's will'. A number of governments instructed their bioethics committees to review the implications of cloning, or moved to ban cloning or restrict access to funds that would allow cloning research. In reports, various authorities were cited or quoted as expressing their dismay and disgust at the prospect of human cloning. In one, 'US bans cloning of humans for five years', President Clinton expresses his response to the findings of the ethics commission which he asked to review the legal and ethical ramifications to cloning: 'One unanimous conclusion has emerged: attempting to clone a human being is unacceptably dangerous to the child and morally unacceptable to our society.' Some articles also included responses from the Catholic Church. For example, in one article a cardinal is reported as describing the idea of human cloning as 'morally repugnant', and as saying that 'all sorts of frightening possibilities can lurk behind these issues' (*The West Australian*, 5 March 1997: 9). Another reported that 'Pope John Paul 2 implicitly condemned research into cloning when he warned on Sunday against carrying out "dangerous experiments" with life', and 'criticized those who "trample on human dignity for the sake of power and money with abuses of all sorts"' (*The Australian*, 4 March 1997: 6). No articles expressed support for human cloning, and no individuals or groups were reported as defending human cloning, although some commentators suggested that cloning adult cells could allow people to 'grow' their own spare body parts. Further, none of the early reports at least presented evidence to suggest that human cloning experiments were under way or imminent. However, many reports expressed the view that human cloning was not only possible but was likely to occur in the near future. The underlying assumption was that since the technology now existed it was inevitable that it would eventually be used. This assumption was probably reinforced by newspaper reports, appearing soon after the announcement of Dolly, that Wilmut, the leader of the research team, had informed a British parliamentary committee that 'human clones could be created in less than two years' (see, for example, Hawkes and Rhodes, 1997: 15).

In the face of widespread public fears about human cloning, and efforts to outlaw cloning research in a number of jurisdictions, many scientists began to make extensive use of the media to defend and explain their work. The torrent of articles on cloning after Dolly makes considerable reference to the views and predictions of scientists, who extol the medical virtues of cloning research, and emphasize the distinction between 'therapeutic cloning' – implicitly seen as 'good', useful, and legitimate – and 'reproductive cloning' – seen as 'bad', dangerous, or illegitimate. As Lee Silver (1998) observes, many scientists who work in the field of animal genetics and embryology were dismayed by all the attention directed at their research, as were those associated with the biotechnology industry, who had most to gain in the short-term from animal applications of cloning technology. Polls undertaken in the United States in the aftermath of Dolly suggest that their fears were not unfounded. These indicated that two out of three Americans considered cloning of animals to be morally unacceptable, and 56 per cent said they would not eat meat from cloned animals. Not surprisingly, politicians sought to distance themselves from the achievement, while scientists attempted to play down the possibility of human cloning (Silver, 1998: 92). A number of prominent scientists who were quoted in the media about their views on human cloning took the opportunity to reassure readers that human cloning was either not possible (or not viable) or served no useful purpose. On the other hand, many scientists, as well as other authorities, expressed concerns that an outright ban on cloning would stifle useful applications, particularly medical applications, such as the cloning of spare body parts. In the aftermath of Dolly, commentators frequently extolled the virtues of the 'acceptable' applications of cloning, which were contrasted with its 'unacceptable' application in human cloning. The views of Wilmut, in this regard, were given extensive press coverage. In one article, published in *The West*, Wilmut was reported as telling a US Senate hearing that 'cloning humans would be unethical and inhumane', and that: 'His group would welcome any efforts that could be made on an international basis to ban human cloning before it occurred.' It went on to note that 'he urged that new laws should preserve opportunities to take advantage of advances in gene manipulation', and that he 'told the Senate sub-committee ... that outright legislation against cloning humans could severely hamper progress towards gene therapies for Parkinson's disease, cystic fibrosis and other diseases' (*The West Australian*, 15 March 1997: 40).

Scientists have been found to draw such distinctions in the attempt to counter what they see as public concerns about the implications of genetic research, particularly its eugenic implications, and to defend an image of geneticists as responsible and ethical professionals (see Kerr *et al.*, 1997, 1998c). Efforts by the scientists who are quoted to explain and justify their research, and to reassure readers of its benefits, are largely absent in the gene discovery stories described above. Articles such as 'Cloning comes of age – just in time', subtitled 'The effects of cloning on the ageing process ... are a big leap forward' (Goldberg, 1998), 'Made to order', subtitled 'Embryo cloning may soon be used overseas to create body parts or cure diseases', (Smith, 1998a), 'Cloners consider our wants and needs' (Lunn, 1998), 'Childless may demand cloning' (Debelle, 1998), 'Scientists urge cloning for spare human body parts' (Woodford, 1999:), 'Grow a new limb using your own cells' (Robotham, 1999), and 'Mad scientist image distorts clone debate' (Amalfi, 1999b) highlight the medical possibilities and benefits of cloning research and serve to reinforce the boundary between 'responsible', potentially useful research and 'irresponsible', potentially dangerous research.

One article, 'Send in the clones', published soon after the announcement of Dolly, offers a detailed account of the medical benefits of cloning human organs, citing case study scenarios, in order to underline the ethical dilemmas inherent in the use of cloning technologies (Smith, 1997: 36). The reader is assisted in understanding 'how Dolly was developed' through a large accompanying diagram, which overshadows the text. The article cites the views of two scientists, one of whom (Dr Ian Wilmut, the 'leader of the team that created Dolly') reassures readers that, despite the absence of laws prohibiting human cloning in many 'high-tech societies', 'most scientists believe human cloning will never be carried out'. The question of 'where to draw the line' between 'good' or legitimate research and 'bad' or illegitimate research is raised in a number of articles. The article 'Cloners consider our wants and needs' opens with: 'Cloning research could lead to genetic restructuring that cures HIV, Parkinson's disease and even quadriplegia, but where do we draw the line and who draws it?' It then goes on to say that: 'If gene technology is allowed to move into more mundane genetic anomalies such as baldness, flat feet or hairy backs, just how far are we from creating a world of supermodels and superhunks?' Again, Wilmut is cited, saying that 'the potential for good medical outcomes from his cloning research "far outweighed the bad"' (Lunn, 1998: 5).

The generally positive images of genetics and geneticists portrayed in the print news media would seem to have been threatened by public perceptions of human cloning. Underlying fears about scientists, science and its products, epitomized in the image of Frankenstein's monster, surfaced in stories about the dangers of unregulated cloning research and 'mad scientists' creating new diseases and threatening human diversity. In a number of articles it is evident that scientists have sought to distance themselves from and discredit Richard Seed, who is portrayed as a 'mad' scientist. For example, he is described by a scientist quoted in one article

('Organ-farming potential heads case for cloning') as 'clearly unhinged' (*The Australian*, 21 January 1998: 10), and by another ('Maverick will clone his wife') as 'crazy and a nuisance' (Smith, 1998b: 11). Public concerns about cloning underline the contingency of public trust in science and medicine, and the importance of positive media portrayals in maintaining the moral integrity of practitioners (Daniel, 1998: 218). The good news stories about cloning portrayed in the media help reaffirm the positive image of genetics and the integrity of genetic researchers, and leave the impression that cloning research can have significant medical benefits.

Conclusion

During a period in which a burgeoning number of new genetic 'breakthroughs' are being reported in the news media, it is crucial to understand both what research gets coverage and how information is portrayed. The chapter argued that by 'framing' issues as they do – by selectively presenting some themes, facts and claims, and not others – the media is likely to exert a powerful influence on public definitions of genetics and its applications in prevention and treatment. Much genetic research of potential significance for treatment and prevention may never be reported in the news, and hence never constitute a subject for public debate and policy, while that which gets reported is likely to be portrayed in ways which reinforce genetic reductionism (Sarkar, 1998). As the above study suggests, the research that does get news coverage tends to focus on single gene disorders and to portray genes as 'causes' of disease. Research is depicted in generally positive terms, suggesting that findings can offer hope for new treatments, tests, or (less often) preventive strategies. There is little negative reporting of genetic research; for example, its potential dangers or high costs relative to public benefits. Although ambivalence about genetic research and its applications is evident in some reports, particularly those dealing with cloning in the aftermath of Dolly, as argued, this has not greatly disturbed the positive overall portrayal of genetics and its applications. Indeed, widely expressed concerns about human cloning arguably have provided the opportunity for scientists to use the media to articulate the value of genetic research by drawing boundaries between genetic research that is seen as 'good', useful and legitimate, and genetic research that is defined as 'bad', dangerous or illegitimate. There is rarely mention of the influence of non-genetic factors and 'multifactorial' interactions on disorders, or questioning of the goals, direction, methods, or value of genetic research. Information that may affect people's evaluations of the research and its significance, such as the commercial interests supporting the research, the influence of polygenetic or non-genetic influences on disease, subsequent disconfirming data, or other experts' critical evaluations of findings, are also largely absent from reports. The absence of such information is likely to offer a powerful constraint on public discourse about genetics and its benefits and risks.

This emphasis and these lacunae in news reporting on genetics and its applications are perhaps not surprising when one considers the processes, described above, which underlie the construction of news about science and technology. Journalists' reliance on single sources of information and on the experts themselves for information and opinions limits the coverage of issues and perspectives. As indicated, scientists have a vested interest in highlighting the benefits of their work, and may emphasize particular diseases and their 'causes' as part of a persuasive strategy to convince people to focus on certain therapies or approaches. The biomedical conception of genetic disease, whereby disease is seen to be a product of a genetic 'defect', governs news media portrayals and reinforces the view that 'quick fixes' and personal risk management strategies, rather than broad social structural and environmental solutions, are needed to prevent illness or restore health. This is not to say that the media presents a single view on genetics and its applications, and offers no scope for multiple interpretations and contestation. As mentioned, we reject a number of widely held assumptions about the 'mediation' of science and technology in general, and about how 'the public' responds to media messages and images. In particular, the notion that scientists produce knowledge, which journalists then make digestible (i.e. 'popularize') for a relatively passive, uncritical, unitary 'public', cannot be sustained. The science 'popularization' model, and the view of subjects as relatively passive, uncritical 'consumers' of information, need to be replaced by a more complex understanding of the interactions between the media and science and between the media and its diverse publics. However, the consistency of the portrayals described in this chapter is likely to strongly shape the agenda for debate and action, especially where alternative information is scarce or absent. We contend that media portrayals constitute an important element of a cultural context shaping how people think about and respond to the new genetics and public health. In the next chapter we examine another important element of this context – genetic counselling – which, as will be explained, is predicted to play an increasingly important role in facilitating people's decision-making in relation to their own genetic risk.

Chapter 5

Facilitating autonomy

The discourse of genetic counselling

Alan Petersen

Assumptions about the 'new genetics' and its potential to transform health and 'empower' 'consumers' are nowhere more clearly articulated than in the rapidly developing area of genetic counselling. In recent years a growing number of writers have expounded the importance of counselling for facilitating autonomy in decision-making before and/or after genetic testing, especially in reproductive decisions but also in treatment and life-style decisions in the case of so-called 'adult-onset' disorders. Genetic counselling is a relatively new profession, which is predicted to play an increasingly important role at the interface between scientists and 'consumers', in both the communication of the risk information arising from genetic research and in offering support to those who are confronted with the attendant choices and dilemmas. This alone makes it an important area for analysis in its own right. However, studies of genetic counselling and its social impacts will be of relevance not just to genetic counsellors or counsellees, since the issues are gaining a broader significance as more and more information about the genetic basis of disease is generated and provides the foundation for decisions in health care. As Clarke argues, the problems that now arise in genetic counselling and its impact on families with common genetic diseases will soon become commonplace in primary health care and medical practice (1997a: 192–3). It is therefore crucial to expose and critically appraise the assumptions that underpin genetic counselling and guide its practices.

In this chapter, we focus on a number of key premises of genetic counselling as these are articulated in the professional literature, and explain some of their implications and limitations in practice. As we explain, despite increasing evidence of the difficulty, if not impossibility, of realizing the ideals of genetic counselling – value-neutrality and 'non-directiveness' – apparent to many practitioners themselves, these ideals continue to be promoted both within and outside the genetic counselling profession. Starting from the assumption that individuals are essentially autonomous and should be 'free' to make their own 'informed' decisions, counsellors have repeatedly emphasized the neutrality of their practice and their role as impartial 'decision facilitators'. In the process they create a distance between themselves and 'the public' whom they seek to serve, and deny the values that inform their practice and the diverse constraints on 'free choice'. The assumptions and language of genetic counselling, we conclude, need to be rethought, and greater recognition needs to be given to the power relations and regulatory implications of counselling. We begin by making some observations on recent trends in the development of genetic counselling and on the broader historical and social contexts shaping its ideals and practices.

Genetic counselling in a historical and social context

As textbooks on genetic counselling explain, the ideals that inform genetic counselling – specifically value-neutrality and 'non-directiveness' – began to be articulated in the early post-World War Two period. However, the development of genetic counselling as a discrete area of professional knowledge and practice has occurred mostly since 1970. Although the first genetic counsellors were medical doctors and researchers, genetic counselling is less and less confined to a particular discipline or area of professional practice. In recent years there have been numerous calls for the expansion of genetic counselling services, and for a broader range of professionals, notably from the primary care area, to undertake counselling. With rapid advances in human genetic research, as a consequence of the HGP and other human 'gene-mapping' initiatives, there is expected to be a shortage of counsellors in the coming decades (Rapp, 1999: 60). Currently, genetic counsellors are drawn from diverse professional groups, including those with medical and non-medical backgrounds, with training and registration requirements varying between countries. Obstetricians, clinical geneticists, genetic nurses, social workers, and specialized counsellors have in recent years offered, and may all currently offer, genetic counselling (British Medical Association, 1998: 127; Kenen, 1986: 175). Despite this diversity of professional contributions, genetic counselling has evolved as a highly feminized area of professional practice. As Rapp observes, as genetic counselling developed it was considered that 'female qualities' like empathic listening seemed especially appropriate. In the US only about 5 per cent of graduates of genetic counselling programmes (usually a two-year masters) are men, and many of these are employed in administration (Rapp, 1999: 56, 60).

Apart from an expected shortage of genetic counsellors, it is also predicted that GPs in primary care will take a major responsibility for counselling patients in coming years and for referring them to other specialists (Check, 1995; Gill and Richards, 1998; Harris, 1998: 337). In the view of the British Medical Association (BMA), GPs are in an ideal position to recognize the likelihood of genetic disorders and initiate discussions about these with patients, since their role is to elicit family histories and monitor the health of families (BMA, 1998: 120). As the recent BMA publication *Human Genetics: Choice and Responsibility* explains, there is growing public awareness of the part played by genes in the incidence of disease and of the possibility of obtaining genetic tests to clarify aspects of one's future health prospects and those of one's children. Thus, increasingly, people are turning to GPs for help in understanding the implications of genetic data and in seeking referral to specialist genetic services. GPs are likely already to know about the backgrounds and dynamics of families, and providing information to assist people with 'informed' decision-making is seen as consistent with the GPs' values and priorities (1998: 120–1). The trend to focus on efficiency in health care, to develop accurate definitions of diseases to predict their clinical course and to choose optimal treatment, it has been suggested, will mean that genetic information will comprise an essential part of future clinical practice (Bell, 1998: 619). The adoption in clinical practice of 'patient-centred' longitudinal health records (see Chapter 1), with the probable inclusion in the future of a growing amount of information derived from genetic testing, points to an acceleration of the move towards what has been termed surveillance medicine (Armstrong, 1995). As genetic testing becomes routine, identified common diseases with a genetic component are likely to include most of the conditions encountered in medical practice. In other words, the very distinction between 'genetic information' and 'non-genetic information' is becoming increasingly artificial (BMA, 1998: 122). In light of these trends and probable future scenarios, some writers have called for the teaching of genetics as an integrative discipline at all stages of professional education, with an emphasis placed on the value of this knowledge to practice (see, for example, Hayflick and Eiff, 1998).

The recent emphasis on the provision of genetic counselling services, and their extension into primary health care in particular, have occurred during a period in which there has been a radical redefinition of citizenship rights and responsibilities. In the post-welfare era, characterized by the winding back of state provision of social services and the promotion of an entrepreneurial culture, the emphasis is on sovereign citizens, who are expected, as part of their obligations of citizenship, to take greater responsibility for managing their own relationship to risk. The dominant approach of genetic counselling – 'non-directiveness' – dovetails neatly with current social ideals such as respect for 'autonomy' and 'reproductive choice' (Wingerson, 1998: 255). With this shift in world view, there has been a broadening of the concept of social citizenship, with a greater emphasis on 'duties implied by rights', which goes beyond the level of the immediate family, the present generation, and the nation state.

The assumptions and language of this new form of citizenship are reflected in the recent literature, including an article which explores the 'legal and ethical issues in genetic testing and counselling for susceptibility to breast, ovarian and colon cancer' (see Dickens et al., 1996). As the authors of this article note, autonomy demands that individuals have a right to be 'adequately informed'. Specifically, their 'decision must be fully informed to the legal standard', and information should be given 'to enable the patient to come to a decision with an adequate knowledge of the risks associated with accepting, rejecting or postponing genetic testing'. However, subjects can only be fully informed if professionals fulfil certain specified duties. In particular, if they are aware of an individual's genetic risks ('in light of family history, for example'), they 'have a duty to inform the patient without being asked'. Professionals have a 'duty to discuss the availability of genetic testing' and, 'unless the physician has been informed of a patient's transfer to another practitioner', they have a duty 'to follow the patient, within reasonable limits, with new information affecting the interpretation of a genetic prognosis and with information about relevant new tests'. Furthermore, they 'have a duty to explain the risk of false-positive and false-negative test results and the uncertain implications of results' (Dickens *et al.*, 1996: 814). Underlying this language of rights and duties is a view of the subject as an independent rational decision-maker who weighs up all available information on risks and arrives at a rational decision, and of information as value-free (albeit changing). However, autonomy is viewed not as a natural given but as an achievement that demands that the subject be fully 'informed' about their susceptibility to risk and about available options, the assumption being that more genetic information will create more choice. (For elaboration on these points, see Petersen, 1998a: 64–6.) In genetic counselling, an understanding of autonomy as 'freedom to act unhampered by external authority' has been elevated to a position of priority, so that it becomes the single guiding principle of practice (Hepburn, 1998: 40).

The 'non-directive' approach

Counsellors seek to facilitate autonomous decision-making through the use of an approach that has been described as 'non-directive', borrowing from the 'non-directiveness' advocated by Carl Rogers in his work on client-centred therapy (Clarke, 1997a: 180). As a contributor to a recent textbook on genetic counselling explains, 'adherence to a nonprescriptive (often referred to as "nondirective") approach is perhaps the most defining feature of genetic coun-selling' and 'stems from a firm belief that genetic counselling should – insofar as is possible – be devoid of any eugenic motivation' (Walker, 1998: 8). Genetic counsellors' deep-seated fears that they will never escape the legacy of the eugenic period have led them to continually reiterate in training sessions and in their professional literature the importance of taking a value-neutral, 'non-directive' stand in counselling. In Wingerson's view: 'There is no one in all of medicine that talks more about value-neutrality than genetic coun-selors' (1998: 254). Questionnaire studies of genetic counsellors undertaken in many countries indicate that the majority of profes-sionals subscribe to the notion of 'non-directiveness', with important exceptions such as phenylketonuria (PKU), where there is seen to be the possibility of preventive action (BMA, 1998: 129–30).

Despite the significance of 'non-directiveness' to contemporary genetic counselling, its meaning, and that of its dualistic oppo-site 'directiveness', is very often left undefined in the professional literature. This is the source of some confusion in discussions since, as Clarke notes, the terms apply to both the broader social context and to the minutiae of the interactions within the counselling session (1997a: 192). Significantly, when it is defined, 'directiveness' is usually equated with coercion, as in the ethical code adopted by the American National Society of Genetic Counselors (1992) and the *Code of Ethical Principles for Genetics Professionals* (1996) (BMA, 1998: 128). The enunciation of such ethical codes reflects the concern of professionals to distance the practices of genetic counselling from what are viewed as the coercive, unethical practices of eugenics. In recent accounts of the goals of genetic counselling, writers have sought to emphasize counselling's 'patient-' or 'client-centred' focus and its role in facilitating individual autonomy or 'choice', which is often distinguished from the broader goal of social 'improvement'. This is clearly evident in an account of 'the objectives of genetic counselling', which appears in the 1998 BMA publication *Human Genetics* referred to above:

> The goal of genetic counselling is to support individuals and families to make choices with which they feel comfortable. In Britain, the service is patient-focused. The practice of UK genetic centres is to emphasize the importance of informed individual choice while bearing in mind the needs of other people in the family who may need to be informed about the implications for them. This focus is very different to that adopted in some countries, such as China, where an overriding preoccupation is the 'improvement' of the population.... The BMA shares the view of many geneticists in the UK that elimination of abnormality within society should not be seen as part of their core aims. High quality and accessible genetic services may well lead to fewer births of infants with some conditions, but this should be seen as an incidental side-effect of service provision. The BMA emphasizes that distance should continue to be maintained between the client-centred focus of genetic counselling and the public health focus on disease. The effectiveness of genetic counselling and genetic services must not be evaluated solely in terms of incidence figures for genetic diseases.... From a practical perspective – and more importantly from an ethical perspective too – funding for counselling and other genetic services

must not be linked to the reproductive decisions of families and individuals.

(1998: 128–9)

Angus Clarke, a UK medical geneticist who has written extensively on the process of genetic counselling, also points to the 'client-focus' of counselling, emphasizing the need for the professionals 'to listen to their clients, to explore their present understanding and their questions and concerns'. According to Clarke: 'The ethos of genetic counselling ... is for the clients to set the agenda, and the first element of genetic counselling must therefore be listening' (1997b: 169–70). (He also notes in this article that this has proved difficult to achieve in practice.) And, in another article, which is co-authored by Clarke, it is noted that 'the ethos of genetic counselling ... is for clients to set the agenda' and that 'the first element of genetic counselling must therefore be listening' (Clarke et al., 1996: 465). As commentators frequently note, respect for the 'client's' autonomy means that counsellors need to eschew paternalism of expert advice and recommendation, in favour of a 'nonjudgemental' and 'supportive' relationship. Biesecker, for example, argues that counsellors need to assist 'clients' to 'maintain control over information about their life and relationships' and remain 'sensitive to the client's needs, health and spiritual beliefs, and cultural norms' (1997: 110–11). This emphasis on 'listening' to 'clients', 'sensitivity to the client's needs', etc., appears to be democratic. However, it denies the inequalities of power between the counsellor and counsellee, and the ways in which counsellors may set the agenda for interaction and control the process of communication, particularly through the use of language (see below).

Most definitions of the objectives of genetic counselling identify the collection and provision of, and assistance with the comprehension of, information – the medical 'facts' – along with post-counselling support, as central elements of counselling practice. This can be seen in a widely cited definition of genetic counselling, adopted by a committee of the American Society of Human Genetics in 1974. The definition refers to genetic counselling as 'a communication process' involving, among other things, 'an attempt by one or more appropriately trained persons to help the individual or family ... comprehend the medical facts, including the diagnosis, the probable course of the disorder, and the available management' (Jackson, 1996: 21). Similarly, the BMA in its outline of the components of genetic counselling notes that genetic counselling includes 'providing information about the condition, its inheritance pattern, and its management', 'giving information about reproductive options', and 'giving information about predictive options' (BMA, 1998: 124). If decision-making is to be 'free' and 'properly informed', it is assumed, then people should be presented with all the relevant medical 'facts', so that they can weigh up all the options and arrive at the 'best' course of action.

This focus in genetic counselling on the adoption of a value-free, 'non-directive' approach, while seen as definitive of contemporary genetic counselling, has not always been an explicit professional goal. In the early years of the twentieth century in the United States, the first 'genetic counselling' centre at the Eugenics Record Office at Cold Spring Harbor (founded in 1910) proffered highly directive advice as to whether to marry or not to marry or reproduce. In line with the eugenic emphasis of the period, counsellors offered premarital, preconception, and postconception hereditary advice with a view to the future of the gene pool as well as the health of the future offspring of their clients (Kenen, 1986: 174; see also Walker, 1998: 2–3). Even in the supposedly post-eugenic period after World War Two, counselling has often had a directive goal, 'telling people what they *ought* to do for the sake of society and their family's future' (Wingerson, 1998: 254). While counsellors during the early post-war period advocated patient self-determination, many geneticists also openly supported eugenic goals. The importance of eugenics to geneticists during the 1950s can be seen in the statements of avowedly 'non-directive' geneticists; these reveal that parents were encouraged not to reproduce in cases where there was believed to be the potential for producing children with 'undesirable traits' (see Resta, 1997). As Resta explains:

> Although they [geneticists] criticized eugenic *programs* that were based on racism and coercion, geneticists still felt that eugenic *goals* were compatible with the goals of genetic counselling. Nondirectiveness was a reaction to the methodology of eugenics, not its principles.
>
> (Resta, 1997: 256; emphases in original)

In the late 1940s and 1950s, when few diagnostic tests were available, counselling was limited to offering families information, sympathy, and the option to avoid child bearing. For the most part, geneticists assumed that 'rational' families would want to prevent births of children with genetic disorders or disabilities (Walker, 1998: 3). As recently as 1972, in the Federal Republic of Germany, when genetics counselling centres were introduced it was argued that: 'The most important task of the genetic counselling centres is to reduce the births of handicapped children within the limits of our possibilities' (Beck-Gernsheim, 1995: 93). And in at least one article originating from the United States in that year, genetic counselling was described as 'preventive medicine' (see Leonard *et al.*, 1972: 437). However, over the last few decades, genetic counsellors have, for the most part, sought to avoid the language of eugenics, and to distance the 'newer' genetics from the eugenics movements of the past from which it evolved, by employing notions of value-freedom and non-directiveness (Brunger and Lippman, 1995: 152; Rapp, 1988: 144; Walker, 1998: 4).

Key features of the 'non-directive' approach

The following account of the 'accepted principles of genetic counseling', which appeared in the edited book *Genetic Responsibility: On Choosing Our Children's Genes*, published in 1974 during a period in which genetic counselling was beginning to professionalize, articulates central features of what have come to be widely identified as key elements of the 'non-directive' approach:

> We try to give a balanced understanding of the nature of the medical problem, its severity and variability, how successful treatment has been, and whether prospects for improved methods of treatment can be foreseen. We indicate the degree of confidence we have about the accuracy of the diagnosis, which family members are affected, and on what facts the diagnosis is based. We give an estimate of the recurrence of risk in numerical terms, expressed both as likelihood of another child becoming affected, and likelihood of him or her being unaffected. We inform the family about availability of prenatal tests for their condition, and when applicable we describe the procedure to them. We include information about the empiric risks that all couples have of bearing a child with birth defects (3%). Our policy is to try to avoid being directive, emphasizing that the information is for their benefit, but that they have the right to ignore it. Usually we do not tell them what other couples in

their situation have done, and when asked we urge them to arrive at their own decisions. We do not ask at the counseling interview whether they have made a decision. When it seems indicated, however, we enquire whether they wish to be directed to family planning services, adoption agencies, or to special facilities for their child.

(Hsia, 1974: 49)

As this reveals, estimations of risk, and the science upon which they are based, are seen as essentially neutral, while the counsellor is portrayed as the impartial, disinterested 'decision-facilitator', who seeks to present a 'balanced' understanding of *the* medical problem. Although there is no pretence that the counsellor is able to provide all the answers, or that diagnoses are completely accurate (in fact the passage hints that, in some cases, they may not be), there is no acknowledgement in this passage of the inevitable selectivity in the presentation of 'facts', and of how the broader social context and the power relations between the counsellor and counsellee shape portrayals of risk. Risk assessments may be presented by the counsellor as either a percentage (e.g. 10%) or as a ratio (1 in 10), which is likely to affect the way in which the information is interpreted by the counsellee. The manner of presentation, and hence reception, of risk information will be shaped by a variety of factors, including the particular setting in which the information is communicated to the client, the broader ideological and policy context, the extent of educational and cultural differences between the counsellor and counsellee, counsellors' expectations about how the information is likely to influence their clients' behaviours, and prevailing notions about acceptable and unacceptable risk.

The 'non-directive' approach assumes that foreknowledge of a statistical risk of developing a genetic disorder permits *better* decision-making on the part of patients/'clients', the unstated expectation being that people will take the necessary evasive action; usually termination of pregnancy. Furthermore, despite counsellors' frequent rhetoric about 'the patient' or 'the client' being not just the presenting individual but the whole family (which might include the foetus), in the case of reproductive decisions it is usually taken to be the mother or potential parents (Hepburn, 1998: 36–7). In the view of some writers, such as Hepburn, the right to 'self-determination' is seen to take precedence over the right to protection of the child, as enunciated in the 1959 United Nations Declaration on the Rights of the Child (1998: 41). As Hepburn explains, genetic testing and genetic counselling reflect a new set of priorities in health care, whereby 'an urge to alleviate suffering is gradually being transformed into a demand that abnormality be eliminated' (1998: 37). The very process of identifying some characteristics, with a view to ensuring that they are not expressed, requires that one counts some abnormalities as unacceptable. The use of genetic testing to select future progeny involves value judgements about what makes life worth living, and thus is inherently discriminatory and eugenicist. Against 'the right to know' about one's genetic risk, some disability organizations have claimed a 'right to abnormality' (Hepburn, 1998: 39). If genetic counsellors were to respect this right, it is argued, genetic counselling would include prenatal information on the social meaning of disability, and what it means to bring up a disabled child, rather than focus just on genetic risk. (See Chapter 7.)

Efforts to promote autonomy

Although imparting information is seen as central to the non-directive approach, as genetic counsellors have come to recognize, this is not sufficient to promote autonomy. While in the early years of the professionalization of genetic counselling (1970s) the main emphasis in counselling was on the communication of technical information and the quality of that information, more and more the emphasis has been placed on *how* that information is understood and acted upon (Kenen and Smith, 1995: 118). In other words, if autonomy is to be achieved, the 'client' must be assisted ('empowered') to become a competent decision-maker:

> Just presenting information does not necessarily promote client autonomy. To succeed in empowering individuals to cope with a genetic condition or risk, or to make difficult decisions with which they can live, the counselor needs to encourage clients to see themselves as competent and to help them anticipate how various events or courses of action could affect them and their families. This cannot be done without knowing something of their social, cultural, educational, economic, emotional, and experiential circumstances. A client's

ability to hear, understand, interpret, and utilize information will be influenced by all these factors.

(Walker, 1998: 8)

In the effort to better 'know' their 'clients', genetic counsellors have proposed new models of counselling, including the 'life history narrative model', to reveal information such as patients'/clients' beliefs about inheritance or the extent to which they feel 'prone' to a genetic disease or feel others in the family are 'prone' to a genetic disease (see Kenen and Smith, 1995: 120). This is not to say that counsellors have come to view the patient/client as a unique and vulnerable person. As Brock (1995) points out, the value placed on non-directive counselling and autonomy reflects the ethos of science, which emphasizes objectivity and universality, and the separation of the scientific mind (the knower) from that which is to be known (1995: 155). In getting to 'know' their 'clients', counsellors reinforce the boundary between themselves and the objects of their enquiry, and reduce the possibility for understanding the unique circumstances of each individual. The context of counselling, which privileges expert knowledge over lay knowledge, leaves little scope for challenging scientific constructions of genetic risk and for reducing the social distance between the counsellor and counsellee.

The use of the term 'client', rather than 'patient', as counsellors' preferred term of address, is consistent with the notions of autonomy and non-directiveness. The term 'client' emphasizes the subject's capacity for independent decision-making, and their readiness to put information to use, whereas 'patient' suggests passivity and diminished capacity for independent decision-making (Brock, 1995: 158–9). It implies that subjects, rather than counsellors or other experts, are the initiators of the interaction and maintain control over the counselling situation. However, counsellors recognize that the context of counselling may thwart the realization of these ideals and that decision-making may need to be facilitated through the pursuit of particular strategies, such as 'scenario-based counselling':

> The clients' questions may focus on the diagnosis or prognosis of the condition being considered, or on reproductive risks and options, or on other issues. The structure of the genetic counselling service is clearly important in deciding whether or not the client's concerns will be heard, in turn deciding whether or how a client's concerns will be addressed ... for some clients,

there is the facilitation of decisions – scenario-based decision counselling – that helps clients to consider the practical and emotional consequences for each of the different possible outcomes of any reproductive or testing decisions that confront them. Finally, there is the provision of ongoing support where this is appropriate.

(Clarke *et al.*, 1996: 465)

'Barriers' to communication

Genetic counsellors have long recognized that there are 'barriers' to the effective communication of risk information, and hence to the achievement of client autonomy. From the very early years of the genetic counselling profession, these 'barriers' have been seen to lie largely at the level of the individual psyche, and to involve either some psychological impediment or individual failure to absorb or retain information. For example, in an article published in 1972 in the *New England Journal of Medicine*, which was based on an interview with parents whose children suffered from genetic conditions and who had undergone genetic counselling, a number of such 'barriers' were identified. These were: 'denial, based on emotional conflict' (10 per cent of the families were found to be 'handicapped in this way'); 'lack of grasp of probability' ('due partly to differences in IQ, education and special experiences' and failure to 'achieve competence' in 'probability comprehension'); and, 'lack of knowledge of genetics and human biology'. 'Evidently, the substratum of biologic knowledge possessed by many parents is inadequate to support the information imposed upon it by the counselor' (Leonard *et al.*, 1972: 438). This emphasis on the individual psyche and on individual failure or 'deficit' (i.e. 'lack of knowledge' or 'failure to retain information') continues in many recent discussions about problems in communicating genetic information (see, for example, Chapple *et al.*, 1995; Evans *et al.*, 1994; Rona *et al.*, 1994). Genetic counsellors have tended to adopt a deficit model which assumes that subjects are ignorant of, or incapable of understanding, risk assessments and the science upon which they are based, and therefore need to be educated or counselled further to overcome the deficit (Petersen *et al.*, 1999: chapter 4). This deficit model is widely deployed by experts in discussions about public understandings of science and is one method of reinforcing the authority of science during a time of acute public scepticism about science and its claims. It denies the importance of lay perspectives on genetics, and the fact that people take up scientific knowledge according to how relevant it is seen to be to their lives (Kerr *et al.*, 1998a: 43). Given the pervasiveness of this deficit model in genetic counselling, it is hardly surprising that genetic counsellors have often defined the counselling process in terms of psychotherapeutics, or as part of 'psychological medicine' (see Hecht and Holmes, 1972: 464). In this view 'the counselor is engaged in a complex psychodynamic process that involves the lessening of denial, the relief of guilt, the lifting of depression, the articulation of anger and, gradually, rational planning for the future' (1972: 464).

Counsellors have recognized that the information they convey has emotional and psychological impacts, and that they need to exercise 'sensitivity' in its communication. Whether the testing is seen as 'presymptomatic' (that is, undertaken by those with a family history of a disorder that might only manifest itself in later life and who wish to discover whether or not they have inherited the gene) or undertaken as part of a woman's or couple's strategy of risk management before embarking on a pregnancy, people who learn that an illness in their family has a likely genetic basis are believed to 'need help with coping'. As one author notes, 'they may feel shell-shocked, bedevilled by feelings of guilt, and suffer a profound loss of self esteem and any sense of purpose in their life' (Pullen, 1990: 47). The range of responses to risk information identified in the recent genetic counselling literature includes: 'grief' ('for the loss of normality and the threat of illness'); 'blaming' the partner (if the illness is seen as inherited from only one parent); 'anger'; 'despair'; 'anxiety'; feelings of shame and 'survivor guilt'; depression, and suicidal thoughts (Macdonald *et al.*, 1996; Marteau and Croyle, 1998; Pullen, 1990: 47–55). With the recent focus on the 'psychosocial and affective dimension in counselling', the expectation is that 'an effective counselor will be attuned to affective responses and be able to explore not only clients' understanding of information, but what it means to them, and what impact they feel it will have in their respective social and psychological frameworks' (Walker, 1998: 8).

Limitations and implications of 'non-directiveness'

What we have described are the ideals and norms of genetic counselling, at least as counsellors themselves have articulated them in the professional literature. The 'non-directive' approach is a principle embraced by all professional bodies, despite growing concerns among practitioners about the difficulty, if not impossibility, of realizing non-directiveness in practice. Although there is little research documenting what counsellors describe themselves as doing, or what they actually do, during the counselling process, there has been some acknowledgement in the professional literature of variation in 'directiveness' of counselling style between professional groups, and between geneticists of different nationalities (Michie and Marteau, 1999: 105). There is also evidence to suggest that a substantial number of counsellors are inattentive to the issues that worry counsellees, and that the former may influence the thinking of the latter about certain things, such as risk magnitudes (Michie and Marteau, 1999: 105). Unfortunately, the professional literature provides few insights into how counsellors may set the agenda in counselling practice and limit the contributions of counsellees. However, a growing body of critical scholarship has pointed to the constraints on 'non-directiveness' posed by the broader ideological and policy context and the power relations between counsellors and counsellees (see, for example, Bosk, 1992; Chadwick, 1993; Clarke, 1991, 1997a, 1997b; Rapp, 1988, 1999). This work could be seen to undermine professionals' idealized portrayal of genetic counselling practice and raises questions about the implications of counsellors' continuing promotion of the ideal of non-directiveness.

Constraints posed by the broader policy context

As some geneticists and counsellors themselves have recognized, the consumer-oriented model in prenatal genetic counselling, whereby individuals are left to make their own decisions, often conflicts with broader policy goals, which focus on measures of efficiency and define 'successful' prevention in terms of termination of the pregnancy. Angus Clarke, for instance, notes that 'it is impossible to maintain a sincerely non-directive approach to counselling about a disorder whilst simultaneously aiming to prevent that disorder' (1991: 999). As Clarke explains:

> I contend that an offer of prenatal diagnosis implies a recommendation to accept that offer, which in turn entails a tacit

recommendation to terminate a pregnancy if it is found to show any abnormality. I believe that this sequence is present irrespective of the counsellor's wishes, thoughts or feelings, because it arises from the social context rather than from the personalities involved – although naturally the counsellor may reinforce these factors. Thus the Holy Grail of non-directive counselling is unattainable, because the counsellor's conscious or even unconscious motives are irrelevant: the offer and acceptance of genetic counselling has already set up a likely chain of events in everyone's mind.

(Clarke, 1991: 1000)

In this article Clarke confesses his unease in dealing with clients who are faced with making decisions about the termination of a pregnancy, especially when they want the child who has been diagnosed with a genetic disorder that does not cause serious medical problems, such as Turner's syndrome. As Clarke explains: 'I resent being obliged, as I often feel that I am, to be economical with the truth in discussions with families who have already terminated a much-wanted Turner's syndrome pregnancy, and strive to avoid adding to the sadness and guilt that they already feel' (1991: 999). In the professional literature, it is uncommon to find comments that are as reflective and questioning as these about the non-directive approach, and that acknowledge the inherent conflicts between broader policy goals and the ideal of client autonomy. Although many individual geneticists and counsellors have acknowledged problems with realizing non-directiveness in practice and have expressed reservations about adopting non-directiveness as a professional ideal, few writers have offered a systematic and critical appraisal of the ideals and practices of genetic counselling. Others, particularly philosophers, sociologists and anthropologists, who are not constrained by counsellors' professional commitments and ideologies, have undertaken most of the detailed analysis and critique.

Ruth Chadwick, a bioethicist, has drawn attention to the common ideological underpinning of the recent emphasis on efficiencies in health care and the focus on autonomy in genetic counselling. Her article is a response to an earlier article by Angus Clarke, in which he raises concerns about the use of measurements of efficiency in medical genetics units based on the number of terminations performed as a result of genetic counselling (see Clarke, 1990). As Chadwick points out, 'the outcome measure proposal comes from the same stable, politically speaking, as belief in autonomy as a political value' (1993: 44). As Chadwick notes, the political ideology behind this measure of efficiency brings 'freedom of choice' into the service of the promotion of self-reliance. That is, 'being autonomous, rather than meaning self-determining, comes to mean standing on your own two feet, so that a rationalization is provided for cutting services while apparently upholding freedom of choice, even though in fact the cuts diminish choice' (1993: 44). In Chadwick's view, autonomy should not itself be seen as the objective because there might be arguments for limiting choice in this area, and, rather than focusing on decisions made (i.e. terminations), a more appropriate measure of success would be 'the extent to which individuals feel that they have been helped by the service' (1993: 45).

Constraints posed by the process of communication

Others, drawing on the findings of qualitative research, have emphasized how the process of communication in genetic counselling undercuts counsellors' formal commitment to 'non-directive' counselling, and reinforces medico-scientific definitions and power relations. Rayna Rapp's (1988, 1999) long-term anthropological study of prenatal diagnosis and the genetic counselling process in the United States is particularly insightful in this regard. As Rapp has found, the language of genetic counselling, employing statistics and medical terminology, limits the quantity and quality of information that a counsellor provides, and 'miscommunication as well as communication, silence as well as conversation, characterize a genetic counseling appointment' (1988: 146). In their efforts to communicate a 'threshold' of information (for example, the concepts of chromosomes and genes, the idea of heredity, and/or the risk of a birth defect involved in any pregnancy and the increased risk of disorders associated with childbearing later in life), counsellors tend to overlook social experiences and the meanings for clients of such things as birth, pregnancy, parenthood and disabling conditions (1988: 147–50; see also 1999: 78–102). As Rapp explains, genetic counsellors are bilinguals, in that they are raised in one language community but have acquired science as a second language. While this applies to many health care workers, 'not all speak a dialect of science as resolutely specialized, statistical, and rapidly evolving as do members of the genetics community' (1999: 62). Furthermore, counsellors attribute specialized meanings to words and terms that appear to have common sense ones. Terms such as 'positive family history' and 'uneventful pregnancy', and concepts such as 'reassurance' and 'ethnic background', hold specific meanings in counselling discourse. For instance, 'ethnic background' has nothing to do with community traditions, but rather marks certain populations as being 'at elevated risk' for specific diseases. These specialized meanings are reinforced in the routines of counselling interactions, where counsellors seek to convey a quantum of 'essential' information, such as information about risks and about the availability and nature of amniocentesis (1999: 62-3). In a UK study, involving an analysis of the transcripts of new genetic counselling consultations, Armstrong *et al.* (1998) similarly found that counsellors' adherence to a routine agenda and almost exclusive use of closed questions served to reinforce counsellors' control of the process of communication. Although clients were seen to offer 'resistance' to this process, by presenting their own 'limited knowledge', this did not disturb the opening routines of the genetic consultation, which were tightly managed by the counsellor and were oriented to locating the client within a 'genetic map' (1998: 1655).

In his ethnographic study in a paediatric hospital, Charles Bosk observed that the ideals of value-neutrality and 'non-directiveness' were frequently breached in genetic counselling practice. Genetic counsellors shaped the way information was presented to prospective parents so as to influence private risk assessment and decision-making. Influence over clients' decisions was seen to arise from the construction of the risk statements which genetic counsellors use to frame alternatives. Firstly, risk statements are comparative in that counselling aims to help people understand their own risks in relation to those of the normal population. Secondly, counsellors frame risk statements in ways that imply what a reasonable and responsible person will do with the information. As Bosk argues, statements 'were framed so that patients could either appreciate the seriousness or the triviality of the problem' (1992: 29). These conclusions are reinforced by the findings of another study, by Brunger and Lippman (1995), based on interviews with genetic counselling students and counsellors, exploring 'how they experience and manage, in practice, the tensions between the ideology of nondirectiveness and the acknowledged reality that one can never be truly nondirective'. As this study showed, although counsellors espoused the ideal of 'non-directiveness' and emphasized the need to present clients with a standard package of facts, counsellors acknowledged that 'in the actual practice of genetic counselling, different individuals *do* need different information' and that 'this led, in consequence, to the constituting of different "facts" to different folks' (1995: 156; emphasis in original).

Constraints posed by 'clients' desire for 'direction' and by different professional contexts and disorders

Finally, some writers have argued that it is difficult for counsellors to remain wholly neutral or 'non-directive' when clients seem to *want* advice or direction (see Beck-Gernsheim, 1995: 93; BMA, 1998: 131; Geller and Holtzman, 1995: 105; Marteau *et al.*, 1994: 867). As Beck-Gernsheim explains, 'they [the clients] feel helpless and probably expect to be relieved of some of the moral and psychic burden of difficult and conflict-laden decisions' (1995: 93). Available evidence suggests that the expectation of advice, and will-ingness to provide advice, is likely to vary across situations, and between health professions. Different professional contexts and different genetic conditions imply different degrees of autonomy for both clients and professionals. In one recent questionnaire-based study in the UK, obstetricians were found to be more directive (i.e. more likely to counsel towards termination) than clinical geneticists and genetic nurses following diagnosis for a foetal abnormality. (The professionals were presented with 17 conditions, varying in severity, age of onset, and type of disability.) The researchers suggest that these differences may be related to differences in training and clinical experiences, and that patients can perhaps more readily be seen as autonomous in the clinical practices of genetics than in the clinical practices of obstetrics (Marteau *et al.*, 1994: 867). In another study, involving focus groups with primary care physicians in the United States, all participants believed that many clients want direction, and some believed that opinion seeking on the part of patients was a sign of trust in the physician. Participants not only thought the goal of 'non-directiveness' was unrealistic, but many saw it as irresponsible, arguing that, if they believed illnesses had family patterns, they had a duty to warn parents about future pregnancies. On the other hand, 'some who were opposed to abortion admitted to framing information about the option of abortion so as to discourage it' (Geller and Holtzman, 1995: 104).

General practitioners, who, as mentioned, are expected to take an increasingly central role in genetic counselling, are especially likely to be 'directive' in their practice and to favour this approach in certain circumstances. As Peter Rose (1999) notes in *Practical Genetics for Primary Care*, GPs may find it more difficult than counsellors to be 'non-directive' since they often know the patient, are involved in their ongoing care, and so, to some extent, will live with the decisions. Despite the move towards a 'patient-centred'/'non-directive' approach, much of primary care involves doctors advising patients 'what to do', or at least influencing their decisions about a course of action. Furthermore, the time constraints of general practice consultations increase the pressure to be 'directive' (1999: 79–80). The BMA acknowledges the problems of achieving 'non-directiveness' in practice, at least in relation to reproductive genetic counselling and, in fact, suggests the use of a 'directive' approach in some cases. As is pointed out in the BMA's *Human Genetics:* 'Direction can be subtle and appear almost as provision of information, such as telling patients what people in their position have chosen' (1998: 130). However, in the BMA's view, this is not necessarily a 'bad' thing since: 'If non-directive support for patient choice were the norm in all aspects of health care, health professionals could end up supporting decisions that are plainly harmful.' Indeed, it is suggested that: 'Counsellors can point out to patients when the latter appear to be choosing in a manner inconsistent with their own values or in a way that they may later regret' (1998: 130–1).

> Even if it ['non-directiveness'] were easily achievable, the provision of dispassionate, impersonal information is not always what many patients want, and genetic counselling recognizes this. It is likely to be less problematic to provide more help when the decision is not about the very sensitive area of reproductive choice. When individuals have to deal with a lot of uncertainty, as in testing for breast cancer mutations, many claim they do not want simply a menu of choices with informa-

tion about each but rather support and guidance about what health professionals would choose for themselves or their families if faced with similar dilemmas. With decisions such as those concerning prophylactic cancer treatment, there is often a fine line between helping people weigh up what testing means for them and supporting them in a way which could be seen as directional by providing reassurance or reinforcement when they decide. Such help and reassurance in those contexts where it is clearly the patient's desire is entirely normal, whether provided by a genetic counsellor or a GP.

(1998: 131)

However, despite the BMA's acknowledgement of the difficulties of realizing 'non-directiveness' in practice and of the fact that patients may desire 'direction', it continues to promote the 'non-directive' approach as 'the general aim of genetic counselling'. It suggests that the relevance of the approach should continue to be emphasized in training, and that 'the extent to which counselling is non-directive should be assessed and monitored' (1998: 131).

Conclusion

Taken as a whole, the above evidence casts doubt on a number of key premises and claims about genetic counselling; namely, the value-neutrality of genetic information and of the counselling process, the ability of individuals to exercise unconstrained 'choice', and the relationship between information provision and 'empowerment'. The assumption that the relevance and significance of genetic risk information is transparent to 'clients'/'consumers' and is independent of sociocultural contexts and of the power relations existing between counsellors and counsellees is increasingly difficult to sustain. Despite this, the view that the genetic counsellor's role is limited to that of information provision and the offering of post-counselling 'support' and that 'choices' are essentially 'private' matters continues to inform debate about the role of genetic counselling and arguments for the increased availability of counselling services. It is noteworthy that, notwithstanding the growing emphasis on the expansion of genetic counselling services into primary health care, where 'directiveness' rather than 'non-directiveness' has traditionally been the norm of professional practice, the notion that counsellors should avoid offering their views or 'direction' continues to be strongly promoted. This apparent concern to distance genetic counselling from what are seen as the coercive practices of eugenics has served to obscure fundamental problems with the 'non-directive' approach, and has arguably restricted debate about the broad regulatory implications of the expansion of counselling services into a growing number of professional areas.

Genetic counselling practice is underpinned by, and reinforces, a view of health as a commodity that can be 'purchased' and 'consumed' like any other commodity in 'the market'. In this view, the individual consumer is seen as responsible for the care of the self by seeking out appropriate 'treatment' and 'support', or by undertaking prescribed preventive action or risk management. This denies the diverse sociocultural constructions of 'health' and 'illness', and the influence of economic, political, and social conditions on people's physical, emotional, and social wellbeing or levels of 'risk'. The concept of the self as autonomous and rational, and as primarily motivated by considerations of personal cost-benefit (e.g. avoidance of disability) and the search for the 'quick fix', overlooks people's diverse backgrounds, experiences, and 'ways of reasoning', as demonstrated, for example, by Rapp (1999). Those who are seen not to follow the above 'ideal' model of rational decision-making are liable to be labelled as suffering a 'deficit', and as therefore requiring education or psychotherapeutic intervention, a response that (as mentioned) has been evident in the history of genetic counselling. In their calls for the expansion of the provision of genetic counselling services, particularly into the primary health care arena, professionals may unwittingly contribute to the blaming of individuals for problems that are largely beyond their control.

The consumerist model of health care is justified on the grounds that it will offer people more 'choice'. 'Consumer' demand and the 'right to know' about genetic health and risk, it is claimed, are the primary motivating forces behind the recent proliferation of testing for common and not-so-common genetic disorders. In the US, DNA tests are available for thirty to forty of the more commonly inherited disorders, including cystic fibrosis, susceptibility to some types of breast cancer, fragile X syndrome, Huntington's disease, and Duchenne muscular dystrophy (Golden, 1999). The supposedly 'demand-driven' provision of a growing number of genetic tests and of genetic counselling diverts attention from the commercial forces and changes in social welfare and health care priorities that underpin and reinforce the genetic world view. (See Chapter 2.) Although professional groups like the BMA seek to differentiate between the goals of genetic counselling and public health (see BMA, 1998: 129), there is growing pressure on practitioners and 'consumers' alike to maximize uptake of services for the sake of 'improved health'. Some writers have indeed suggested that a new 'user-friendly' eugenics has emerged, or is emerging, spurred not through political ideology but through the operations of the market and as the collective product of individual decisions (see, for example, Rifkin, 1998: 128–9). In the professional literature of genetic counsellors there is little apparent recognition of how the language of consumerism reinforces a particular world view and associated set of priorities, dispositions, and actions. Although there is evident growing dissatisfaction with conventional 'outcome measures' of genetic counselling (e.g. recall of information and alteration of reproductive plans or behaviour) among at least some practitioners (see, for example, Clarke, 1997b), there has been no fundamental challenge to the dominant individualistic and consumerist model of health that informs practice.

The need to evaluate the aims and regulatory implications of genetic counselling has become urgent in light of recent calls to widen the network of experts involved in genetic counselling and to forge multidisciplinary collaborations between GPs, paediatricians, obstetricians and other specialists who act as 'gate-keepers' to genetic counsellors (see, for example, Kenen, 1997; Kenen and Smith, 1995; Harris, 1998). These calls have occurred during a period in which there has been increasing demand for new tools of surveillance, including improved methods for recording genetic data, as well as more extensive use of 'genetic family registers' to identify and track 'at risk' family members (see, for example, Harris, 1998; Malinowski, 1994). With the growth in the number of conditions subject to genetic testing and counselling, and the development of improved means for collecting, storing and accessing genetic information (e.g. the use of 'patient-centred' medical records), there is increased potential for surveillance and regulation to occur. As the focus on genetic health intensifies, the notion that genetic counsellors can, and should, be value-free and 'non-directive' will become ever more difficult to sustain. Growing demands for genetic testing and genetic counselling will create pressures on health planners, medical geneticists, and counsellors to make difficult decisions about who is to be tested and counselled and what constitutes an acceptable or unacceptable level of risk. In other words, counsellors will be required to become *more* directive. There is the danger that an increasingly directive genetic counselling practice may occur behind the smoke screen of the rhetoric of value-neutrality and non-directiveness. Appeals to this rhetoric may serve to conceal the expansion of new, insidious forms of control based on assumptions about human genetic makeup and difference – a possibility that is recognized by various groups. In the final chapter we explore how both opponents and supporters of new genetic technologies have responded to, and have sought to influence the development of, these technologies. Before turning to that discussion, in the next chapter we broaden our focus to examine the global context within which the new genetic technologies are emerging.

Chapter 6

Global genes

Robin Bunton

From its outset the development of the 'new genetics' has been firmly situated in the international arena and intimately linked to global economic processes and cross-national industrial formation. If the twenty-first century is, as Rifkin (1998) argues, the 'biotech' century, it is also a globalizing century. The biotechnologies are being seen, in the West at least, as promising sources of profit and economic development, and as a means of solving the nutritional and health needs of the world's expanding population. Chapter 4 outlined the 'bio-fantasies' in Western media representations of genetic science. The promise of 'breakthroughs', cures and increased control of disease is highlighted in these accounts. The 'race' for 'the complete gene map' by the Human Genome Project and Celera Genomics has been portrayed as a dash for scientific certainty and progress, bolstering a belief in the idea of scientific progress and the rational control of the natural world. This 'progress' is also being seen as global progress, despite acknowledged fundamental challenges and difficulties presented by the new genetic science and despite public concern for some of its consequences.

The development of the new genetics is intimately linked to economic concerns and the profit motive. New types of partnership and alliance between scientists and entrepreneurs have emerged in the last twenty years or so that have led some to speak of a 'new paradigm' of scientific practice in which the interests of science and capital coincide. Information and life sciences, it is argued, are coming together to manage genetic information as a 'raw resource' for the new global economy (Rifkin, 1998). Biotech and bioscience companies are growing in power. They operate globally and are constructing a 'bioindustrial complex' which seeks biotechnological innovation as a new means of capital accumulation (McNally and Wheale, 1998). Starting in the 1970s, transnational corporations and venture capitalists invested in genetic engineering firms. Commenting on the development of the American gene therapy industry, Martin (1995) has observed that:

> Like many other areas of biotechnology, almost all the dedicated gene therapy firms were founded by leading academic researchers, many of whom were instrumental in developing gene transfer techniques. The firms were initially set up with the help of entrepreneurs and venture capitalists, often as a way of commercialising the techniques being developed by scientists in a particular research institution.
>
> (Martin, 1995: 160)

Major interest from pharmaceutical firms such as Monsanto has led to the biotech market becoming one of the more important areas for speculation and investment.

> It is clear that neither the scientific nor commercial development of gene therapy has occurred in existing producers of therapeutics, but has required the creation of a series of new firms to drive this process. This is perhaps explained by the fact that gene therapy operates within a radically different conceptual paradigm from traditional pharmaceuticals.
>
> (Martin, 1995: 157)

This chapter will consider some of the implications of the new genetics for health and welfare in an international perspective. Throughout most of this book we have focused on the implications of the new genetics for the nature of social relationships and health in Western societies, and the ways in which ideas of citizenship, governance and responsibility are being changed by the new means of risk surveillance and regulation that the new genetic technologies afford. Here we want to turn attention to the ways in which global relationships are being changed across state boundaries and some possible global consequences for health.

Globalization and health

Globalization has received considerable attention in recent years, in medicine and the social sciences. At its simplest globalization refers to the increasingly interconnected nature of the world and the ways that events in one part of the world, perhaps thousands of miles away, will have an influence on local events. The concept is used in different ways but usually denotes the growing spread of a capitalist world system and its integration with systems of trade, communication, transportation, patterns of urbanization, cultural influence, and migration throughout the world, and involves the movement of people, information, symbols, capital, commodities and organisms (Kearney, 1995; Zielinski-Gutierrez and Kendall, 2000). Globalization refers, then, to economic and sociocultural processes that can have a profound effect on health and the social relationships that underpin health care systems.

We can identify both the globalization of health and disease states and the effects of globalization on health and disease. The interconnected nature of the world has led to observations that there is a convergence of disease patterns between 'advanced' and 'developing' countries, possibly reflecting globalization. Increased economic linkages, transportation, changes in the environment and urbanization are said to be responsible for the increasing numbers of persons in both higher income and 'developing' countries being affected by non-communicable diseases such as ischemic heart disease, unipolar major depressions and cerebrovascular disease, and road accidents. This disease process is no longer the preserve of higher-income countries, and the predictions of the Global Burden of Disease (GBD) suggest a shift away from the 'epidemiological divide' that for so long has distinguished countries of the North and South. Communicable diseases still persist, however, and account for significant differences in the distribution of death that still exist between established market economies and the former socialist economies as well as the 'developing' world, and some communicable diseases will become more important, especially HIV/AIDS (Murray and Lopez, 1996). In parts of sub-Saharan Africa, for example, HIV/AIDS is responsible for reversing increases in life expectancy achieved in the last two decades.

The idea of 'epidemiological polarisation' (Mosley et al., 1993) is useful in understanding the divergent trends in health under conditions of globalization. Increasing chronic disease and entrenchment of infectious disease can be found among lower-income populations in the developed and the developing world. Mechanisms such as the rapid diffusion of new technologies are allowing improved health among subsectors of the population. It is also likely that economic dislocations accompany these processes in ways that marginalize and impoverish other sectors of the populace, 'either through new exposures to pathogens, the creation of new disease enhancing environments, dislocations of land tenure and traditional food supplies' or through other effects (Zielinski-Gutierrez and Kendall, 2000).

Although pandemics and imported diseases have been in existence since the sixteenth century (Diamond, 1997), increased migration, transport and trade have introduced new levels of uncertainty into the microbial world. Predictions would suggest that the total burden of disease in the world will see little change in the next decade or so, though the relative burden of disease is likely to shift so that the poor in all regions will suffer more than those on higher incomes from infectious disease (Murray and Lopez, 1996; Zielinski-Gutierrez and Kendall, 2000). Similarly, the general health benefits of globalization are likely to be distributed unevenly.

Globalization has been primarily a project restricted to only a few countries of Europe and North America during the twentieth and twenty-first centuries. Fuelled by capitalism and technological development, globalizing processes carry with them the cultural values of the West, including 'acquisitive individualism' (Lasch, 1991) and technological optimism. Developments in enterprising genetic technologies are, similarly, Western led, with major investment in North America. The industry at present and in the future is likely to involve largely Western finance and likely to be Western led with little real investment for the South. The major 'gene-technology-rich' seed corporations, such as Monsanto, are primarily Western led.

The negative effects of globalization processes relate not simply to the globalization of disease but also to the effects of associated economic and sociocultural processes, often a result of Western dominance. Globalization would appear to be exacerbating social inequalities and the imbalance of political and economic power between the North and the South. The recent World Development Report (1998) of the United Nations Development Fund pointed to under-consumption as the main constriction on better health for the developing world. In the last fifty years or so the liberalization of trade and the flows of capital have facilitated technological and industrial processes that have concentrated food retailing in the hands of fewer international companies, affording less opportunity for state governments to regulate consumption for health. Similarly, the bioagricultural industry is centrally involved in developments that threaten to overwhelm local production patterns and social structures of small-scale farmers in the poorer countries of the South. In doing so, they are implicated in cultural as well as economic imperialism that may have detrimental effects on health by creating further social and cultural uncertainty and risk.

Accounting for the social impact of the new genetic knowledge and associated technologies must take place within an understanding of the changing global relationships surrounding health. There are direct health risks attached to the new therapeutic techniques or newer genetically modified organisms. There are also less direct effects on health resulting from changing economic and cultural processes produced by the new biotechnological industrial complex and its influence on health and welfare. The new genetic techniques are culturally inscribed with the values of Western health-care systems and make often unseen value impositions. These aspects are apparent when we consider the development of patents for human and plant genes, and the development of GMOs in agriculture.

Patenting and the commodification of health

The development of patents for human genes has been a contentious issue and provoked much public debate in recent years. The debate frequently reflects ambivalence about the privatizing effects of new genetic science and technologies in relation to health. There has been a remarkable growth of patent applications in recent years. Public and private institutions, for instance, filed over 9,0000 claims on 127,000 human genes or partial human gene sequences in 2000, which included nine applications for patents covering 38 genes of the human eye (*Guardian*, 15 November 2000). There are different patenting rules across the world, and the US patenting rules and philosophy are more relaxed than those of Europe. The USA's Patent and Trademark Office and the European Patent Office are also subject to the World Trade Organization's Trade-Related Intellectual Property Rights agreement. The US biotech lobby led the campaign to claim 20-year patent protection on human, plant and animal gene sequences in a series of court judgements in the early 1980s. The US Patent and Trademark Office granted the first gene patent in 1975 to Stanford University and the University of California rights to Boyer and Cohen's gene-splicing technique, paving the way for a rapid growth in investment. Boyer himself founded Genentech in 1976, and the company was floated on the stock market in 1980. Venture capital was sought and by the mid-1980s there were about 500 free-standing biotechnology firms engaged in genetic engineering, which were joined by a number of other large chemical and related industrial firms. In 2000 the US boasted upwards of 1,300 firms, Britain 450, and there were around 800 small and medium enterprises in Europe (*Guardian*, 15 November 2000). Growing at around 20 per cent per annum, the industry represents one of the most sought-after investments on the market. It would appear that the rush for patents continues to grow. The European Patent Office currently has a backlog of 15,000 biotechnology patent applications.

Reporting of this growth has been critical of a certain 'gold-rush' mentality and, in Europe at least, there remain some legal challenges to the Patent Offices and the European Parliament's condoning of patents. German Greenpeace, for example, has campaigned to challenge the European Parliament's 1998 Patenting Directive and drive for profit. The language of these challenges is indicative of the critique of the commodifying of genes. Accusations of 'bio-pirating', 'prospecting', 'bio-colonialism' or even 'vampirism' indicate the moral distaste for patents. Some of these objections emerged in opposition to the Human Genome Diversity Project (HGDP) based at the universities of Yale and California. The HGDP was founded to prepare cell lines and DNA from blood, hair or saliva samples taken from populations that have been geographically isolated or have a distinct culture and language. These were referred to as 'Isolates of Historic Interest' (Roberts, 1993). The stated purpose of HGDP was to study the genetic basis of disease susceptibility. The material was to be shared with scientists worldwide for research on human history and biology. The information was to be used to construct genealogical trees and to answer the question: How much do individuals vary from the composite 'reference' sequence that will emerge from the Human Genome Project? Opposition to this research project came from various quarters and led to the International Bioethics Committee of the United Nation's Educational, Scientific and Cultural

Organization (UNESCO) setting up a subcommittee and holding hearings to represent indigenous peoples and develop international guidelines for the project or similar projects (Randall, 2000). The case made by some aboriginal groups is one that rejects the cultural assumptions of Western scientific research, showing clearly the value-laden nature of genetic science.

Indigenous peoples protested vigorously from the outset of the research programme, and concerns about patenting and commercial exploitation were raised worldwide. Whitt (1998) reports on the reaction of Australian Aboriginal people and quotes John Liddle, the director of the Central Australian Aboriginal Congress:

> If the Vampire Project goes ahead and patents are put on genetic material from Aboriginal people, this would be legalised theft. Over the last 200 years, non-Aboriginal people have taken our land, our language, culture and health – even our children. Now they want to take the genetic material which makes us Aboriginal people as well.
>
> (Nason, 1994, quoted in Whitt, 1998)

Others had raised the question: 'How soon will it be before they apply for intellectual property rights to these genes and sell them for a profit?' (Tauli-Corpus, 1993). Though proponents of the HGDP repeatedly saw such opposition as a 'misunderstanding' of science, the difference between the two perspectives illustrates fundamental differences in philosophy. As Mead (1995, 1996) points out, the Maori translate the word 'gene' as 'iratangata' ('life spirit of the mortals') or 'whakapapa' ('genealogy'). A physical gene is viewed as imbued with a life spirit handed down from ancestors. Genes are part of successive families, communities, tribes and entire nations; that is, they are not the property of individuals and cannot, therefore, be privatized or commercialized in cell lines. The property rights implicit in the patenting exercise are abhorrent to such an ethic, and genetic science exercises such as the HGDP are experienced as theft.

The abhorrence expressed by some aboriginal people reflects fundamental assumptions about the public ownership of certain features of existence. Somewhat similar sentiments were and continue to be expressed by commentators in Western public debate, who see genes as elements of nature and/or life which should not be put under private ownership or control. It has been argued that DNA sequence patents are morally objectionable because patent-based property rights should not be made on 'the building blocks' that make up mankind (Randall, 2000). (A technical point that often accompanies this argument is that patents should only be granted to inventions not based on 'a discovery of nature'. DNA sequences are a discovery of nature and therefore not patentable.) DNA, it is argued, is a part of the 'gift of life' and fundamentally a public good, and should not be subject to private market forces.

Resistance to the commodification of nature and the body are not restricted to societies steeped in traditional religious or non-scientific knowledges, as the recent controversy over the Icelandic health sector database illustrates. International controversy emerged in the autumn of 1998 when Icelandic plans to build a health sector electronic database using the near total Icelandic population as its biological sample became known. Emerging from research initiated in 1994 on genetic aspects of multiple sclerosis, by Harvard clinical neurologist Kari Stefansson and colleagues, the idea of a large sample database was introduced to the Icelandic public when a bill was presented to the Icelandic parliament to facilitate a private/public partnership in the database. Iceland provided a unique opportunity to collect data on a large, relatively isolated and genetically homogeneous population in order to study genetic aspects of common diseases. It was an opportunity for what is being termed 'functional genomics' (Martin and Kaye, 2000) to draw upon genetic samples, medical records and genealogical records to assist in the development of therapeutics. Private finance has assisted, and a private company, deCODE Genetics, has led the study. The preliminary stages of what led to the Iceland Biobanks Act (finally passed in 2000) immediately generated intense public debate among Iceland's scientific and clinical communities, but, in the main, the project was supported by the Icelandic public. Elsewhere public and professional fears of the 'brave new world' consequences of the new genetics emerged, with headline stories such as 'Iceland sells its people's genome' and 'Selling the family secrets'. Fears about the security of anonymity were not helped by the first draft of legislation not allowing people to withhold consent, nor ensuring that medical record data was to be made anonymous.

The Icelandic bill came under criticism from a number of quarters, especially data protection experts. It brought to the surface many of the social and ethical concerns that were referred to in Chapter 5 in relation to counselling. Members of Europe's Data Protection Commission considered that the draft bill would violate several European treaties, including the European Convention on Human Rights (Rose, 2001). The Icelandic case focused broader academic interest on the social and moral issues involved in large biological sample collections. Interest in such projects was emerging in the UK and elsewhere, with strong academic and commercial involvement (Martin and Kaye, 2000). These cases raise some novel and searching questions about the adequacy of regulatory and ethical monitoring bodies.

The intense social and moral debate surrounding these developments relates to the enormous potential of genetics to intensify the commodification of nature and the human body. Such commodification transfers what are considered to be collective or personal qualities and places them in the hands of corporate ownership for private gain. The debate also concerns the commodification of knowledge and the increased use of knowledge and technology in the production process. As Rose observes, the Icelandic case demonstrates the fusion of biotechnology and informatics, creating a new commodity – bioinformation:

> Biotechnology (using informatics) is bringing into existence an entirely new class of information – genetic information – but it is informatics itself which enables old forms of information, the medical records and the genealogies, to be brought into relation with the new, creating a historically new and marketable commodity.
>
> (Rose, 2001: 23)

Rose refers to Shulman's observation that the intensification of patent claims for intellectual property is indicative of this process as a new wealth of nations (Shulman, 1999). This new commodification dates back to the 1980 landmark case of the successful patenting of bacteria designed to eat crude oil, when the US Supreme Court ruling determined that 'anything under the sun made by man' was patentable. Patenting is based upon the principles of transference to corporate ownership (for a time period) of that which was either collective or personal property.

Resistance to the commodification of perceived 'public goods' has been debated previously in relation to health and welfare.

Titmus (1970) described the public availability of Blood Transfusion Services in the UK as a 'gift relationship'. Drawing upon the anthropological work of Lévi-Strauss and also Mauss, Titmus argued that the donation of blood can be understood as an altruistic and collective social act – giving blood to the 'unknown stranger' – made in the face of considerable, modern commercial pressure towards individualized self-interest. Such altruism, he claimed, underlay moral and ethical commitments to welfare systems in the West. Titmus compared the more wasteful and costly American system of selling blood, which also carried higher health risks, with that of the UK, concluding that 'freedom from disability is inseparable from altruism' (1970: 246). Titmus's work on blood, then, similarly identified the anti-commodification phenomena apparent in resistance to the genetic commodification of 'blood-lines'. It would appear that a contra-tendency is developing in relation to the patenting of human genes which supports an increasingly commodified, individualized health care ethic.

The new genetics knowledge and technologies are being intro-duced to health care systems at a point when state support for health and social welfare services is diminishing. The privatization of health and welfare is supported by the promise of genetic regula-tion and the commercializing of therapies. This undermines the notion of health and social care as a 'gift'. One effect of globaliza-tion is said to be the 'hollowing out' of the local state (Robertson, 1992), as matters previously dealt with by state institutions become a matter for the market, the family and newly empowered citizens. Technological solutions are often seen as a means to fill the vacuum left by diminished health and social services with 'hot-line' and 'on-line' support care (Burrows and Pleace, 2000). The promise of the new genetics offers not simply newer, cheaper solutions to health problems but also new high-tech services. The new genetic technolo-gies, then, represent a new commodification of health and health care in a global capitalist system of production that is increasingly intertwined with and dependent upon knowledge and information.

Market forces of late capitalism, it would appear, are increasingly 'knowledge rich' and draw upon information as much as physical 'raw materials' (Castells, 1996). Consumer products, goods and services are becoming impregnated with information, and informa-tion and knowledge are being brought to the service of economies. Increasingly, we live and work within 'economies of signs and space' (Lash and Urry, 1994). In such economies patents and intellectual property rights become more important as they facilitate more opportunities for further commodification. Wealth creation is made possible by the generation of ideas and information. Bio-technoscience relies upon patent law in a process of what Whitt (1998) has referred to as 'bio-colonialism'. Whilst colonialism encompasses a range of economic, social, cultural, political and legal policies and practices, bio-colonialism emphasizes the role of science policy and other means of extracting valued genetic resources and information. 'Discovery' by 'bio-prospectors' or 'bio-pirates' (the terms for a range of geneticists, botanists and other scientists) is largely undertaken in countries of the South to inform research and development in therapeutic medicine development and agriculture. As Whitt points out, intellectual property laws:

> serve as a means of transforming indigenous knowledge and genetic resources into profitable commodities, and of advancing the commodification of nature. For example, the chief of the Global Environment Division of the World Bank, discussing traditional plant knowledge in the Ethiopian Coptic Church, recently proposed: 'Let's screen that knowledge stock [and] explore how it might be commercialized....' Indigenous representatives to the Commission on Sustainable Development have challenged the practice of bioprospecting, and the global imposition of western intellectual property laws.
>
> (Whitt, 1998: 235)

Patenting, then, as a means of attributing property rights, commodifies and privatizes nature. In doing so, life is transformed from a common 'gift' into a private good, and a product for exchange in the increasingly global marketplace. The transformation of nature into commodities, as Karl Marx observed (1967), has profound implications for social relationships. The 'gift' relationship is revealing of social relationships and social values. Titmus (1970) observed how gifts engender ties of 'brotherliness' and obligation. Once nature is commodified as private knowledge, no such obligations remain. When a gift is rendered into a commodity not only is its metaphysical status changed, but also the giver no longer has control over its use. Opponents of such commodification and bio-colonialism regard initiatives such as the HGDP as an assimilative process that threatens to transform indigenous knowledge and value systems as well as the natural world itself. The knowledge, resources and labour of generations of indigenous peoples, without control over their intellectual property rights, is expropriated without material benefit reaching them.

Bio-colonialism on a global scale illustrates the ways in which the new genetic science carries with it cultural inscriptions and the individualizing and privatizing of collectively 'owned' parts of existence. Patented genes are being sought for newer, information-rich, global economic processes. The inscription is apparent also in the types of health care solutions that are being offered by the use of such genetic resources. The biotech companies currently work to a predominantly Western health care agenda and are shaping gene technologies to suit the health care systems of the West. The recent focus on gene therapy emulates previous biomedical techniques, resulting in conceptions of gene therapies as drugs (Martin, 1999). The new technologies may improve current practice, but they are likely to maintain health care within a high-cost, high-tech model that is highly inappropriate for export to countries of the South. Such technologies bolster a particularly Western version of health care that is based upon a notion of health as a commodity to be bought and sold in a largely privatized system. Despite assurances from world leaders, such as the joint statement of the UK Prime Minister Tony Blair and the US President Bill Clinton that: 'Raw fundamental data on the human genome ... should be freely available to scientists everywhere' (Theif, 2000), Celera Genomics and the HGP are led by Western scientists, and the use and development of this knowledge is unlikely to be equal across the globe. By advantaging the richer nations, such technology may further exacerbate the divide between industrialized and 'developing' countries. Globalized modelling of health care in this way is likely to be problematic, reflecting only a one-way, North–South political and cultural influence (Navaro, 1993, 1998). Moreover, if the 'epidemiological divide' continues to be important, then public health initiatives rather than privatized care systems are likely to be more important in the poorer regions, as they will embrace a larger health burden resulting from infectious diseases.

The exportation of Western cultural values via medical technologies brings with it particular challenges. The 'breakthrough' strategies to deal with malaria in the mid-twentieth century were dependent upon new technologies that could transform the environment in many countries (the use of insecticides) and the development of vaccines since the 1980s (NIAID, 1998). The continued use of drugs and vaccines is impeded in many countries by high costs, however, and new technologies can make countries dependent upon the multinational corporations that produce them, often at high costs. In early 2001 an intense international debate took place over the use of cheaper drugs to combat AIDS, tuberculosis and malaria. The European Parliament exerted pressure on thirty-nine drug companies to stop a legal battle to halt legislation that would allow South African imports of cheaper medicines to combat AIDS. Brazil has been seen as the exemplar of the response of developing countries to such health crises, allowing the manufacture of cheap copies of the patented drugs used to combat the HIV/AIDS virus (*Guardian*, 31 March 2001).

It is of course possible that the newer genetic technologies could address the health problems facing 'developing' countries and poorer regions, and issues of environmental manipulation and cheaper vaccine delivery in particular. Such is the promise of some technologies. Research is taking place to develop edible vaccines in tomatoes and potatoes (Whitman, 2000). Such development is likely to take place alongside changes in bio-agriculture, to which we now turn.

GMOs and global processes

GM food or GMOs (genetically modified organisms) are terms that have entered everyday parlance over the last decade or so. Commonly referring to crop plants created or modified for human or animal consumption using molecular biology techniques, these plants are adapted to enhance desired traits such as increased resistance to herbicides, improved nutritional content or enhanced features. The advantage of new molecular technologies over more traditional plant breeding methods is that they are quicker and more accurate. Genetically engineered plants would appear to hold great hope and promise for both profit and environmental improvement, and also possibly for health.

Plant geneticists have isolated genes for drought tolerance that can be inserted into a variety of plants. Modification has also been made to increase pest resistance, herbicide tolerance, disease resistance, cold tolerance and nutritional value. The use of crops for developing medicines is also receiving some attention, such as the feasibility of human antibody production in plants (Russell, 1999). It is possible for genes from non-plant organisms to be transferred into plants and grown. A well-publicized example of this is the use of *Bacillus thuringiensis* (B.t.) genes in corn and other crops. B.t. is a naturally occurring bacterium that produces proteins lethal to insect larvae, enabling crops such as corn to produce their own pesticides against insects such as the European corn borer (http://www. biotechknowledge.com/primer/primer.html). While the science is at an early stage of development, as in the field of human genetics, the promise of such research is both exciting and seductive, and it suggests a number of solutions to global health problems.

Economic advantage is also a fundamental feature of these information-rich commodities. A flavour of the excitement and economic ambition behind potential 'gene-rich' production can often be found in definitions of the field of biotechnology itself, as in the following:

> In a system so dependent on biological processes, modern biotechnologies have truly revolutionary implications. They confer a technical capacity to undertake selective genetic inter-vention in existing forms of life and to create novel life forms. The genetic code can be manipulated and nature refashioned according to the logic of the marketplace. As a result, biotech-nologies have suddenly provided new alternative paths of development for major actors in the food system; farmers and import suppliers, primary processors, final food manufacturers and consumers. It is this crosscutting, polyvalent capacity of biotechnologies which makes them such a potent force in restructuring the food systems.
> (Goodman and Redclift, 1991, quoted in Bainbridge *et al.*,2000: 1)

A sense of economic optimism can be found in scientific reporting of new developments, as in a recent article in *Science* by Guerinot (2000) with the title 'The green revolution strikes gold'. The produc-tion of transgenic crops such as 'Roundup Ready' soybeans, developed by Monsanto, and corn expressing B.t. toxin promises to reduce costs to the farmer by minimizing the application of herbi-cides and insecticides. Perhaps the greatest promise comes from those crops which would serve as better sources of essential nutri-ents, potentially improving regions of extreme poverty. The promise of agricultural biotechnology is taken seriously, with predictions of a world population of 7 billion by 2013 and double that by 2070.

Recent reports of a new 'golden rice' strain are typical of the optimistic claims. Such rice, it has been claimed, could save millions of lives and improve maternal and child health in developing countries by increasing the iron and vitamin A content of the rice grain, as *Science* magazine has reported (January 2000):

> Developed by the Swiss Federal Institute of Technology's Institute for Plant Sciences, [golden rice] could significantly improve vitamin uptake in poverty stricken areas where supplemental pills are costly and difficult to distribute. The International Rice Research Institute (IRRI) – part of the Consultative Group on International Agricultural Research (CGIAR) – is working with the Swiss scientists to adapt the new 'golden rice' to developing country conditions.
>
> (Guerinot, 2000: 241)

Ninety per cent of the world's rice is grown and consumed in Asia, where more than half the world's people and about two-thirds of the world's poor live. Subsequent research has reported that, though 'golden rice' is useful, the amount of rice intake necessary to combat diet deficiency was far larger than those living in poor regions with poor diets could afford.

A potential 'gene revolution' follows closely on the heels of the 'green revolution' which transformed 'developing' economies from the middle of the last century (Spallone, 1992). This revolution may have far-reaching consequences for environments and our economies. The development of commercial agricultural biotechnology has been rapid. Since 1986 around 25,000 transgenic field trials have been held worldwide, 10,000 of these between 1999 and 2000. The global area of GMO crops has increased sharply from 1.7 million hectares in 1996 to 11.0 million ha in 1997, and more than 28 million ha in 1998, representing a fifteen-fold increase (Buttel, 1999). Despite these developments, crop biotechnology is still relatively limited in scope and involves only a few major crops. The US had more than one third of GM soybean acreage and one fifth of cotton acreage in 1999. Argentina and Canada also have a significant GMO acreage and together with the USA accounted for 99 per cent of GMO acreage in 1998. A similar race for patenting licences has occurred in GMO research and development. In 2000 there were 152 applications for patents on rice, covering 584 genes or partial gene sequences. Similar fears of bio-colonialism are apparent in relation to such a rapid rush for intellectual property rights.

Considerable concern has been voiced about the harmful effects of globalization, particularly the shifts in the balance of world agricultural power and the potential harm that the new technologies engender. The financial interests of the world bio-agricultural industry and its ambitious investment in the newer GMO techniques have come under critical scrutiny. The rapid commercialization of biotechnologies in the industrialized world, it is feared, could lead to threats to employment or labour displacement in developing countries due to a change in international trade patterns. Potential bio-substitution of crops or changes in industrial and food processes aided by genetic technologies (Galhardi, 1995) could lead to erratic and uncertain economic processes. Moreover, the 'colonisation of the seed' (Shiva, 1992) could mean that wealthier bio-agricultural multinational corporations come to dominate and control the world food supply. Given the current investment leadership balance, this would mean increased Western dominance over food production, further exacerbating the North–South economic and health divide.

Despite the widely publicized benefits of GMO production and the potential 'revolution' in agriculture and medicines, the public have remained sceptical of the commercial production of transgenic food crops, particularly in Europe. Citizens in the EU and other countries of Europe are more ambivalent about the agrifood biotechnologies than Americans and have strongly supported EU restrictions on the import of GMO products. There is also considerable consumer resistance to GMOs, which has impacted on retailing strategies in Europe. Several large grocery chains, such as the Co-op, Marks and Spencer, Safeway, Sainsbury's, Tesco and Waitrose, under pressure from anti-GMO consumer groups, formed something of a GMO-free consortium in 1999 (Buttel, 1999). Several other manufacturing multinationals such as Unilever, Nestlé and Cadbury Schweppes made similar commitments. Such action puts pressure on US manufacturers, some of which have required their corn and soybean suppliers to segregate GMO crops from their non-GMO counterparts. This action by consumer groups flies in the face of World Trade Organization guidelines concerning non-tariff barriers to trade, which preclude import restrictions that are based on a product having been produced through genetic engineering alone.

Being citizens of some of the richest nations of the world, European consumers can afford to object to the consumption of GMOs in food. Such a luxury may not be possible for many countries in the world, and it may be that GMO crops that are perceived to be a risk to health are exported to poorer regions, maintaining a global trend of risk exportation or transfer found in sales of pharmaceuticals, tobacco and other health-damaging products. A recent Institute of Medicine report has characterized the result of economic globalization as a transfer of 'risk' due to the movement of people, the exchange of toxic products, and the variation in environmental safety standards (Institute of Medicine, 1997; Zielinski-Gutierrez and Kendall, 2000). Globalization has meant that production processes can be located in countries with lower labour and production costs, which often coincide with less regulation of industrial risk factors. Global capital is capable of overriding local systems and forms of regulation that are frequently ill prepared for newer, potentially dangerous, technologies. While catastrophes such as the Indian Bhopal incident are a feature of this, even mundane technologies can be problematic.

> Mundane objects out of context can prove dangerous; for example, the recycling of insecticide and herbicide sacks for the storing of food and seed grains in rural Central America has grave consequences for health. The changes in local economies due to international market influence, a re-definition of local medicine according to cosmopolitan medical standards, and the influx of new risks – social, behavioural and biological – appear to have overwhelmed the local ability to adapt and cope.
>
> (Zielinski-Gutierrez and Kendall, 2000: 87)

The one-sided interconnectedness would appear to allow risks to be exported to other regions. In addition, by placing these technologies in novel settings, newer kinds of risk are likely to emerge.

The health risks associated with genetic modification have been referred to in Chapter 3 – in our discussion of the environment and public health – and include: risks relating to the altered nutritional quality of foods, antibiotic resistance, potential toxicity, potential allergenicity, and more general environmental health threats (Uzogara, 2000). Here we are concerned more with the effects of genetic science and technologies on the conception of health and health care systems globally.

The accusations against the genetic-industrial-agriculture complex are considerable and share much with critiques of the chemical-industrial agriculture typical of the 'green revolution'. Both these forms rely on capital-intensive, externally supplied inputs such as seeds, fertilisers and pesticides. They both involve large-scale 'mono-culture' cropping of uniform plant varieties (Scrinis, 1995). Genetic-industrial agriculture, then, will tend to further reduce biodiversity by replacing indigenous plant varieties with uniform varieties developed by the seed companies. It may create a new set of 'super-pests' as resistances to static plant varieties develop, which will in turn require further chemical and biological pesticides to be developed to control them. A related danger is the spread and proliferation of new genetic traits in other domesticated and wild plants through cross-pollination, for example – a type of genetic pollution. There is evidence that such intensification will result in unsustainable industrial agricultural practices by creating plants that can tolerate degraded or marginal soils, or greater applications of chemical inputs. The culmination of these processes is that farmers will lose independence and self-sufficiency and become more dependent on multinational bioindustrial-agricultural firms. The increased global interdependency may have unperceived political and economic consequences. In information- and technology-rich production processes it is possible to bring together chemical and genetic technologies to further enhance control of the production process. Crops may be designed to match insecticides. The scenario is suggestive of considerable cross-national centralization and control, as Scrinis has pointed out.

> This fusion of agribusiness corporation and techno-science now culminates in the triumph of the logic of the code; in particular, the *genetic-code* of biotechnology, and the *bar-code* of consumer-industrial capitalism. The genetic-code and the bar-code are the means through which ever more aspects of contemporary life are being colonized, commodified and controlled. In this context, it is not unlikely that the fusion of these two codes will ultimately manifest itself in the imprinting of bar-codes on the DNA of genetically engineered organisms, thus securing the corporate ownership and control over the micro-structures of life itself.
>
> (Scrinis, 1995: 38)

The 'colonization of the seed' will achieve a similar shifting of power from public ownership of, often communal, farming to private ownership, which will leave power and greater financial reward in the hands of predominantly Western bio-agricultural corporations. An example of this process provoked international debate over the so-called 'terminator seeds'. The US agribusiness giant Monsanto was developing sterile seed technology. The terminator gene would render seeds produced from a GM crop infertile, meaning that farmers would be forced to purchase seeds each year from the supplier, rather than propagate their own seed stock, as they had for centuries. Monsanto and other biotechnology companies argue that such 'gene protection systems' are necessary to safeguard their huge investments in GM crops. This particular strategy was criticized for its greed and the detrimental effects it would have on farmers and the environment. Monsanto made a public commitment to abandon this line of research in 1999 in an open letter to the Rockefeller Foundation President. The Monsanto backdown on this issue was seen as a major victory by the anti-GM product lobby. The episode highlights the concern about the economic concentration of power in a small number of 'gene-rich' seed companies. There are only seven or so major corporate groups in agricultural biotechnology worldwide, including: Novartis (Ciba Geigy, Sandoz, Northrup King), DuPont/Pioneer, Monsanto/ DeKalb/Holdens, Seneca/Advanta, AgrEvo, American Home Products, and Dow/Mycogen/Elanco (Buttel, 1999). Most of these corporations are involved in agrochemical, seed pharmaceutical and food product lines as well as in crop biotechnology.

Redistributing control in this way is likely to mean a loss of income and power for poorer, small-scale farming in countries such as India. As Shiva (1993) has pointed out, cash cropping can mean that small producers lose ownership of their crop and the cash. The shift from organic and substance farming to capital-intensive, market and cash-crop oriented agriculture will have social consequences such as the undermining of women's traditional roles in food production in many countries of the South (Shiva, 1993). Cash crop production tends to fall under male control and takes away land and resources previously controlled by women.

Patenting law and intellectual property rights cases underpin much of the new GM world order and, as McNally and Wheale have pointed out:

illustrate how the categorisation of the products and the processes of modern biotechnology and genetic engineering as patentable subject matter is producing a global ordering of life forms and social agents which creates and reinforces inequities between the advanced industrial countries and the less developed countries.

(McNally and Wheale, 1998: 304)

McNally and Wheale argue that about 80 per cent of biodiversity is located in the less developed countries, particularly in Asia and South America, that are 'gene-rich' but 'gene technology-poor.' Conversely, the advanced industrial countries are technology-rich but gene-poor. Advanced countries can reap great financial benefit, then, by means of intellectual property rights and the internationalization of patenting. The current state of biodiversity is the result of the work of indigenous peoples who have recognized, protected, developed and utilized its potential. Patents cannot be given *in situ*. Uniqueness is only recognized by the patenting system when extracted, manipulated, characterized, etc. The patenting possibilities of genetically engineered crops greatly enhance the potential for the corporate control of agriculture by large 'bioagropharmachemical multinational companies' (McNally and Wheale, 1998: 314).

Conclusion

By processes of commodification, the introduction of techno-industrial agriculture creates not only biological uniformity but also cultural uniformity, globally. It undermines the small-scale, organic mixed cropping, sustainable farming systems of the many countries of the South. Like the commodification inherent in human genetic developments, gene technology is culturally inscribed. It engenders particular types of social relationship and particular types of production process. This account is suggestive of a rather one-way project of globalization that will reproduce Western notions about health, the environment and nature throughout the world. The new genetic technologies appear as culturally inscribed artefacts that have transformative qualities for those that come into contact with them.

The effects of the globalized marketing of genetics are similar to those of the marketing of fast food. Analysing the success of fast-food franchises such as MacDonald's, Ritzer (1993) points out that more is being consumed than Big Macs. The success of fast food is more than a product success story, it is a characteristic of the progressive standardization and bureaucratization of everyday life brought about by a range of products and standardized production techniques. Products such as cars, education, supermarkets increasingly represent a way of life and a set of 'standardized' values emanating from a single cultural centre. It is emblematic of a particular cultural and economic imperialism. It is, however, a rather reductive account of global processes. It is no longer possible to speak of globalization as a simple process involving the dominance of a single centre over the peripheries (Featherstone, 1995). It is more accurate to conceive of a number of competing centres that struggle for the balance of power between nation states. There are more players in the game. The dominance of Western scientific communities in the development of new genetic industries appears to be promoting one set of interests. Resistance to the genetic science and technologies being pursued can be seen as the presence of other 'voices' or cultural challenges to such impositions. The outcome of struggles over particular technologies, such as the 'terminator' genes or the HGDP, will have far-reaching consequences for the conception of health and health care systems in the rest of the world. In the 'post-genome' era it is difficult to offer firm predictions about the likely direction of change. However, as is explained in the next and final chapter, it is clear that, increasingly, citizens are expected to actively participate in decisions about new genetic technologies and their applications in the advancement of the public's health. Whether the participatory mechanisms that have been developed will allow citizens to significantly influence policies and practices remains to be seen.

Chapter 7

The new genetic citizens

Alan Petersen

In many, if not most, public forums where the impact of new genetic technologies is debated, the voice of the expert tends to be privileged over the voice of the non-expert. Arguments generally polarize around contending professional viewpoints: the new technologies are portrayed as offering either unqualified benefits or, much less frequently, unmitigated dangers for 'the public'. There is often a failure to acknowledge the diverse, and often complex, views and responses of the actual or potential 'consumers' of the new technologies. Further, despite an increasing emphasis on citizen participation in policy in general, there has been little exploration of the opportunities for diverse *publics* to be involved in decisions about the development or applications of the genetic technologies that affect them or are likely to affect them. This final chapter examines the diverse responses of those groups that have been, and are most likely to be, immediately and directly affected by the new genetics, and evaluates recent efforts to involve 'the public' in decisions about new genetic technologies. In the process we hope to unsettle some dominant assumptions about the new genetics, the self, and social relations, and present alternative ways of thinking about and evaluating the impact of new genetic technologies on people's lives and relationships.

The increased attention given to 'genetic literacy', combined with the rapid integration of genetic technologies in strategies of prevention, has enhanced many people's awareness about their genetic health and risk, and given rise to new categories of identity and novel forms of sociality and citizenship. Many people have been identified, and have begun to identify themselves, as being 'at risk' or as victims of a genetic disease or disability, or as carriers of a genetic defect, and have organized to advance or protect their citizen rights as members of a genetic category. Some have formed or joined 'support groups' in an effort to educate the community about genetic disorders, to advance their rights to access to information and to 'informed choice', and to lobby to increase funding for research and improved support services. These groups often work in partnership with public health practitioners and other experts to advance their objectives, and play an active role in shaping research priorities, research funding, and the provision of services. However, others, including feminists, disability rights scholars and activists, and racial and ethnic minority rights groups, have expressed concerns about the potential for the new genetic technologies to erode existing rights, and have organized and lobbied to protect those rights. They tend to be more critical of science and expertise, drawing attention to past eugenic abuses. They are inclined to emphasize the need for social changes to eliminate discrimination and to promote recognition of difference. The emergence of such groups and forms of action attests to the power of the new genetics to shape people's thinking and to transform lives. In the following paragraphs we examine these diverse responses, and finally draw some implications for further work by exploring the social implications of new genetic technologies. First, however, we wish to elaborate on some points about 'freedom of choice' and active citizenship that have been recurring themes in this book.

Active citizenship and 'freedom of choice' in the context of the so-called new genetics

As argued, notions of 'freedom of choice', 'right to know', and 'informed decision-making' pervade writings about 'the new genetics'. By presenting new options, the new genetics is frequently portrayed as a force for liberation, in that it is seen to enhance individual freedoms, which distinguishes 'it' from eugenics, which is conceived as coercive and repressive. Within new genetics discourse, human beings are posited not as passive recipients of expert advice but as *active citizens* who weigh up all the options and decide upon their own course of action. In the case of reproduction, the responsibility for decisions, it is claimed, has been democratized. As Clague expresses it, 'choices are taken by individual consumers', and 'families determine their own genetic futures; they decide which genetic disorders to tolerate' (Clague, 1998: 10). This emphasis on 'freedom of choice' and 'self determination' in genetic decision-making reflects a more general emphasis on active citizenship in many contemporary societies, evident, for example, in public health, welfare, and education (see Petersen and Lupton, 1996; Petersen *et al.*, 1999). In Britain, it was announced in late 2000 that the rudiments of active participation are to be taught via a booklet, *Active Citizenship*, in the National Curriculum for 11- to 16-year-olds from September 2002 (Birkett, 2000: 5). In Australia active citizenship has also been emphasized in recent government policies 'as a foundation stone for a healthy and inclusive community' (Johnson, undated: 2). This emphasis on active citizenship, although generally discussed in public forums without reference to questions of power relations and politics, can be seen as a manifestation of a particular operation of power that has become increasingly widespread in late modern societies.

As Foucauldian scholars emphasize, in contemporary societies, the governance of populations is achieved not so much through repression but through the active participation of 'free' subjects; that is, subjects who are able to exercise their agency without coercion from an external authority. Nicholas Rose notes that freedom has a double-edged character: it is both an ideal, as in struggles against a particular regime of power (i.e. contestation), and a mode of organizing and administering populations that depends upon the capacities of free subjects (i.e. an exercise of power) (N. Rose, 1999: 66). In politics both the Left and the Right subscribe to the ideal of freedom. In the former, the appeal has been to freedom from economic enslavement; in the latter, freedom to compete in the free market, to maximize profit, and (as consumers) to choose between products. What recent scholarship makes clear is that 'freedom' is a historically and socially specific construction that has been deployed by different groups with different objectives, but is always held as a positive ideal. Few people in societies with a liberal democratic tradition would argue against the ideal of freedom – whether freedom *from* constraint or freedom *to* choose. Increasingly, we have come to be defined, and to define ourselves, in terms of our freedoms. Diverse forms of expertise and disciplinary practice, and personal practices of consumption, are addressed to individuals as free subjects, and encourage us to think of ourselves as autonomous and as exercising freedom of choice (N. Rose, 1999: 66–97). Through practices of consumption, for example, individuals are offered ways of living, or a style of life, which promise personal happiness, health, and wellbeing through acts of choice in the world of goods. Similarly, the 'therapeutic' disciplines of psychology and psychiatry encourage us to think of life as a plurality of possible life-styles, and of the self as an object of knowledge that is subject to self-improvement through the application of rational knowledge and techniques (1999: 85–93). The influence of therapeutic thinking is clearly evident in genetic counselling, which, as we noted earlier, is oriented to facilitating 'choice' and individual 'empowerment'. As Rose notes, through such transformations in expertise and practices, 'individuals are not merely "free to choose", but *obliged to be free*, to understand and enact their lives in terms of choice' (1999: 87; emphasis in original).

The idea that power 'acts through practices that "make up subjects" as free persons' (N. Rose, 1999: 95) is very different from traditional conceptions of power as a negative and repressive force. Within these negative conceptions, freedom is imagined as freedom from coercion or domination; a condition in which individuals are not silenced or subordinated by an external power. Arguments against eugenics tend to invoke this negative conception of power. As mentioned in Chapter 2, eugenics is objected to not so much because of its goal (which is broadly similar to that of contemporary public health genetics; i.e. the betterment of population health), but because it involves an exercise of power that is seen to curtail the freedom of subjects. To say that freedom has become a paramount ideal in politics, it should be emphasized, is not the same as saying that people act as fully autonomous (i.e. unconstrained) beings, for freedom is always *regulated* (Rose and Miller, 1992: 174). Both the range of options for action, and the way those options are exercised (the actual decisions), are constrained by the broader economic and social context, including policies which increasingly are based on the criterion of cost-effectiveness. Thus, choices which are seen as unsustainable or to impede the efficient running of the system, and those – such as people with disabilities – who are seen as incurring a cost to society, may be greeted with intolerance (Clague, 1998: 11). As mentioned in Chapter 5, some writers have criticized 'non-directive' counselling on the grounds that it is not possible to be truly non-directive in a context in which values of efficiency and criteria of treatment 'success', generally measured by the number of terminations, are paramount. In this view, the notions of participation and 'freedom of choice' are *harnessed* in the service of cost cutting and the reduction of services, and serve to deflect attention from the social context within which decisions are made. Thus, although the move towards greater citizen participation in the development of science and health policies may modify social conditions for significant numbers of people, at least in some areas of practice there has been minimal impact on public policy or the public agenda (Miringoff, 1991: 127–46). As we will explain below, one of the observations made by critics of new genetic technologies is that the choices that they are seen to offer are often illusory in that they are constrained, and do nothing to alter the conditions that affect the lives of disadvantaged groups.

The ideals of active citizenship, it should be emphasized, are not simply imposed 'from above'. The rhetoric of freedom and participation permeates the language and writings of professionals and non-professionals alike. Public health practitioners, scientists, and lay people all frequently draw on the same discourse of empowerment in discussions about the applications of new genetic technologies, and may work in partnership in an effort to advance this ideal. Specialist genetics education programmes, genetic services, public health practitioners, and genetics support groups have developed, often as collaborative ventures, an array of educational materials and resources, with the aim of promoting people's 'genetic literacy' and their active involvement in the monitoring and management of their own genetic health. The Internet has proved to be an important 'enabling' tool, allowing professionals and lay groups alike to forge networks, to expand citizen involvement and to strengthen links between groups at the national and international level. Indeed, it can be argued that the development of the technology of the Internet has been an essential precondition for new forms of sociality associated with the new genetics. The Internet has greatly facilitated people's access to ideas and to key personnel and institutions. (See, for example, the publications *Technology and Public Participation*, and *Models of Public Involvement*, available on the net: http://www.uow.edu.au/arts/sts/TPP/ and http://www. pip. org.uk/models.htm). Many of the forms of association that have arisen in recent years would have been inconceivable without the networking possibilities opened up by email and the Web. There have emerged new 'virtual communities' of genetics experts and the genetically diseased, disabled, and 'at risk'.

Recent efforts to advance active citizenship in relation to new genetic technologies

Over the last decade or so a growing number of practical strategies have been adopted to advance the ideals of active citizenship in relation to new genetic technologies. Indeed, 'public participation' has been the catch-cry in relation to many areas of science and public policy in addition to genetics, and governments, public health experts, and private sponsors have repeatedly emphasized that not only do citizens have a right to participate but that they have a *duty*. For example, in the UK the importance of 'consumer involvement' in science policy was highlighted in February 2000, when a report of the House of Lords Select Committee on Science and Technology recommended that dialogue with the public should become a normal and integral part of science-based policy-making. And, recently, the UK-based Wellcome Trust has sought to provide a forum to discuss issues of 'consumer involvement' and to inform its own policy in this area through, for instance, hosting meetings involving patient groups, policy-makers, research funders, scientists and representatives from pharmaceutical companies (Bailey, 2001: 6–7). In some cases, laws have been passed to institutionalize participation, with government officials and some businesses sometimes seeking to enhance the extent and intensity of participation in response to evident frustration on behalf of sections of 'the public' (Webler and Renn, 1995: 26). Suggested and tried participatory mechanisms include opinion polls, focus groups, referendums, citizens' forums, future search conferences, citizens' panels (planning cells), citizens' juries, consensus conferences, deliberative opinion polls, and public meetings (Coote and Lenaghan, 1997; Joss and Durant, 1995; Stewart *et al.*, 1994). Through the deployment of such means, the message is conveyed that it is crucial for people to become 'scientifically and technologically literate' and 'be actively involved' in decisions affecting their own health and wellbeing, particularly through the management of genetic risk.

The recent literature on citizen participation expresses growing dissatisfaction with traditional political processes, which are experienced by 'ordinary citizens' as alienating and 'disempowering'. The problem, according to Dienel (1989), is that decision-making has become increasingly professionalized and specialized:

There are signs of a new cleavage between two social classes: the privileged 'decision makers' and the 'administrees', the majority of the population. As can be seen by reading almost any newspaper, the typical reaction to this situation is indifference or aggression. This is damaging to our political system.

(cited in Stewart *et al.*, 1994: 9)

Another commentator, who is arguing for citizen participation in solving environmental problems, observes that traditional decision-making strategies are increasingly recognized as insufficient. Often heavily shaped by scientific analysis and judgement, these kinds of strategies are liable to two major critiques:

First, because they de-emphasize the consideration of affected interests in favor of 'objective' analyses, they suffer from a lack of popular acceptance. Second, because they rely almost exclusively on systematic observations and general theories, they slight the local and anecdotal knowledge of the people most familiar with the problem and risk producing outcomes that are incompetent, irrelevant, or simply unworkable. Citizen involvement in decision making has been widely acknowledged as a potential and partial solution to these problems.

(Renn *et al.*, 1995: 1)

Although the theoretical influences on thinking about mechanisms of participation and their evaluation have been diverse, the ideas of the sociologist Jürgen Habermas have been especially influential in the recent literature. One of the reasons for the popularity of his work is that his theory gives credence to individual autonomy. It is Habermas's view that individuals ought to be free of all forms of domination and that, once free, people are able to enter into social relations that facilitate personal development and the development of society and culture. The emphasis is on critical self-reflection: introspection among free and autonomous beings should be promoted so that they will think about the type of society that they want *before* committing to new social relations. Public participation is the means to realize the critical self-awareness (Renn *et al.*, 1995: 9). Habermas's focus on individual autonomy and his consensual view of society sit well with the neo-liberal views on self and society.

Citizens' juries and other participatory structures, it is argued, seek to redress the so-called 'democratic deficit' by 'enabling' non-professionals to have a voice in the important decisions which affect them. As Stewart *et al.* explain, the aim of citizens' juries and similar mechanisms is 'to foster the habit of active citizenship' (1994: 4–5). Citizens' juries are seen as especially effective for the opportunity they provide for 'informed' deliberation upon issues such as the introduction and use of new technologies, such as genetic technologies. Although they are relatively time-consuming and costly, they are seen as better at tackling complex questions and difficult choices than other models (1994: 90). While this and other suggested mechanisms may be relatively new, the espoused concern to counter the alienating, 'disempowering' effects of the modern bureaucratic form of power is not. Those who advocate the use of such mechanisms draw on a long tradition of thought that counterpoises the imagined small-scale Gemeinschaft (community), involving face-to-face encounters and consensual decision-making, with the large-scale Gesellschaft (society), involving the exercise of impersonal power and representative decision-making (Plant, 1974: 15–22). The use of citizens' juries in the United States and Germany has been justified on the basis of 'bringing some of the benefits of small group, face-to-face decision-making to large scale democracies' (Stewart *et al.*, 1994: 10). Increasingly, citizens' juries and other decision-making mechanisms are seen as a way of overcoming citizen apathy and inculcating a sense of duty and responsibility *as citizens*, linking personal motivations and actions with broader social goals. The problem which citizens' juries seek to address, and their goals and modus operandi, are neatly summarized by Stewart *et al.*

> The ability of ordinary citizens to make difficult decisions in increasingly complex areas of policy is often doubted by experts and politicians. One result is that many citizens feel incapable of making decisions about anything beyond their immediate and personal daily lives, and therefore lack the motivation to become informed about political issues. Thus the split between government and the people widens. The citizens' jury process attempts to deal with such problems. Ordinary citizens meet in a group of manageable size to deliberate on policy issues, rather than delegating this responsibility to others. The face-to-face nature of debates is seen as a way of drawing people into the political process, enabling them to think not as isolated, anonymous individuals, but as citizens, working together via dialogue and consensus for the 'common good' of

society. Because it would be impossible for every citizen to attend a citizens' jury, jurors are selected either at random or to represent society (by criteria such as gender, race and age). This is claimed to enhance their sense of duty and responsibility, since jurors feel they are speaking on behalf of thousands of citizens just like them. Jurors can show competence in their decisions, because they have the time and the motivation to become informed about the issue at stake. This, combined with the opportunity to question politicians and other experts, imbues the jurors with a sense of confidence that they are capable of making complex decisions about their own lives and those of their fellow citizens.

(1994: 10)

In recent years a number of 'experiments' involving new mechanisms of participation have been conducted in response to what is perceived to be citizen disenchantment with the 'top-down' decision-making processes of mainstream politics. Reflecting this trend, efforts have been made to gauge 'the public's' views on new genetic technologies. For example, a citizen jury approach was used in Wales in 1997 to broaden public participation in the decision-making processes surrounding the introduction of new genetic technologies in health care (Dunkerley and Glasner, 1998; Glasner, 2001). During the 1980s and 1990s consensus conferences were used in many countries, including Canada, Norway, Denmark, the Netherlands, Australia and the UK, to enhance the participation of both lay persons and experts in the assessment of new genetic technologies, as well as other technologies (Mayer and Geurts, 1998: 288–9).

Despite the evident good intentions underlying these efforts, a number of commentators are sceptical about the effectiveness of participation as it has been articulated thus far. A major problem, according to Renn et al. (1995), is that: 'Confusion about the goals of citizen participation accompanies every practical application.' Part of the reason for the lack of agreement on goals is that the parties involved tend to define them in ways beneficial to their own best interests (1995: 4–5). While citizens, administrators, stakeholders, and experts may all desire participation, they are likely to have quite different reasons for so doing, and have different ideas about how the process should be conducted (1995: 5). There is no standard procedure for assessing participatory mechanisms. Indeed, commentators are divided about the necessity of assessment, the aims of evaluation, and the appropriate research methodologies (Joss, 1995). Although in some contexts (e.g. Denmark) some such mechanisms (e.g. consensus conferences) have arguably helped shape the use of concrete technologies and the allocation of research funds, they have been of limited value in changing the technological culture or the social dynamics surrounding concrete artefacts (see Cronberg, 1995: 13). In some jurisdictions (e.g. Germany) citizens' juries are regarded as having strengthened representative government through public participation. However, in others (the United States), citizens' juries have been posited 'almost as an alternative to decision-making by elected representatives and have not yet influenced actual political decisions' (Stewart *et al.*, 1994: 52). Some commentators argue that such mechanisms are best viewed as complementing rather than supplanting existing decision-making processes, so as to address the problem of weak democracy (e.g. Armour, 1995: 186; Stewart *et al.*, 1994: iii, 7).

Across virtually all contexts, the question of the criteria of representativeness of the participating group(s) has been the subject of vigorous debate. In the case of the citizens' jury, because it involves so few individuals at any one time, it has been suggested that it can only be seen to represent the community *symbolically* (Coote and Lenaghan, 1997: 91). Since the citizens' jury cannot be precisely representative, it is argued, its decisions should be seen as advisory rather than binding, and as one component in a broader public involvement exercise (1997: 91). Glasner (2001) contends that the lack of representativeness of the 1997 citizens' jury experiment in Wales – particularly as regards well-established ethnic minority groups – has 'largely erod[ed] one of its key democratising principles'. Further, he (2001) notes that such participatory mechanisms are often underpinned by an unarticulated model of expertise that is likely to undercut efforts to involve lay people in decision-making. In relation to citizens' juries, the configuration of the categories of 'lay' jurors and 'expert' witnesses sets the terms for engagement, where experts have the power to set the agenda and define the boundaries of discourse (Glasner, 2001). This occurs through, for instance, the selection of preliminary information made available to lay members and the use of witnesses. When actors are granted an 'expert' status, they are empowered to speak on almost any aspect of biotechnology, regardless of the reason for their participation. Several of the witnesses appearing before the citizens' jury experiment in Wales saw the primary justification for using the citizens' jury approach as educative rather than participative (Dunkerly and Glasner, 1998: 189). The jury model also brings with it a great deal of symbolic baggage, including the notion that there is a neutral reality that can be 'discovered' under strictly objective conditions. This denies the complexity and 'messiness' of the process of policy formation. Despite its symbolism, the citizens' jury inadequately mirrors the ritualistic elements found in the court of law, which establish the legitimacy of the outcomes (Glasner, 2001).

Taken as a whole, such criticisms lead one to question the extent to which lay publics can significantly shape the genetic research and development agenda through such means. Given the powerful commercial interests involved in the development of genetic technologies, and the close connections that often obtain between business and government, it is perhaps overly optimistic to expect that non-experts can exert significant influence over the broad directions of research and development. The limitations of the citizens' jury approach in this regard were powerfully underlined by a recent citizens' jury experiment in India (heralded as 'the South's first citizen jury on GM crops'). Despite Indian farmers' expressed concerns about GM crops, articulated through a citizens' jury, a biotech company (Monsanto) subsequently won approval from the Indian Department of Biotechnology to release its GM cotton on to the Indian market (Wijeratna, 2000: 7). This example suggests that participatory mechanisms such as citizens' juries may serve as a coopting device, giving the impression of a shift in power relations but having no material effect on the final decisions.

While such practical efforts at active citizenship may be judged to have fallen short of the ideals in a number of key respects, it is clear that many people continue to subscribe to the ideals. This is reflected in various groups' efforts to influence decision-making in relation to new genetic technologies. Groups' responses and strategies have been diverse, including those who actively promote genetic research and those who lobby to restrict or regulate the development of genetic technologies. Regardless of their perspectives and methods, however, virtually all groups affirm the importance of participation and 'freedom of choice' as ideals of contemporary citizenship, although conceptions of 'freedom' and of the means by which it can be best achieved vary considerably. In the following paragraphs we examine how people who are affected, or believe they will be affected, by new genetic technologies have sought to realize these ideals, and some of the arguments and strategies that they have deployed.

The new active citizens

Genetic support groups

An obvious example of where citizens have organized to influence decisions about new genetic technologies is genetic support groups. Genetic support groups generally endorse the development of new genetic technologies. Drawing heavily on the language of participation and 'consumer' rights, they emphasize the significance of genetic information to 'informed' decision-making, as well as the need for appropriate support services for members. They demand the *freedom to choose* that is seen to arise from new options created by genetic research and the right to consume new genetic products. They seek to advance their claims by forging links with international 'umbrella' support groups, networking through the Internet and other forums. These groups are formed either by individuals with genetic disorders and their families or by health care providers, such as genetic counsellors, nurses, social workers, and physicians (Mackta and Weiss, 1994: 519). As Mackta and Weiss explain:

> Genetic support group members usually are composed of individuals representing a cross-section of society who have been brought together by a genetic disorder that affects themselves, a family member, or both. Because of the life-long impact of these disorders and the small proportion of the population represented, there is an added urgency motivating people to join the organization. Many of the groups have evolved from a few dedicated individuals working around a kitchen or family room table. Quite a few voluntary organizations operate without staff and function through the hard work of family members and friends. Genetic support groups often supplement the work of the genetics team, including the geneticist, genetic counselor, nurse, social worker, and other specialists. These groups can become strong allies in reinforcing clinical goals.
>
> (1994: 520)

Genetic support groups attempt to influence policies and practices affecting those who have already been diagnosed with a genetic condition. They do this by providing information and suggestions to the professionals, for example about the impact of the genetic disorder on the individual and family, as well as to the parents. They sometimes assist professionals in compiling lists of potential peer-support individuals who can help patients who have anxieties about the new diagnosis of disease in their children or themselves (1994: 520). Information is often disseminated via 'resource books', which include directories of genetics support groups. For example, the *Genetics Resource Book: The Australian and New Zealand Directory of Genetics Support Groups, Services and Information*, produced by the New South Wales Genetics Education Program, contains information on 759 support groups for specific genetic disorders across Australasia (Genetics Education Program, 2000). This publication includes a summary of each of the disorders, a list of resources, and the support groups in each state or territory. It also includes international information and support groups for genetic disorders, details of available services in each of the states and territories, and 'information and fact sheets' pertaining to 'your family health tree', use of genetic counsellors, gene therapy, and the HGP.

During the 1980s and 1990s international 'umbrella' support groups have developed in Europe, the UK, the US, Canada, the Netherlands, South Africa, Australia, and New Zealand (Genetics Education Program, 2000: 144). The Genetic Alliance (formerly Alliance of Genetic Support Groups), formed in 1986, is typical of 'umbrella' groups in terms of its goals, organization and modus operandi. According to its web site, the Genetic Alliance is 'an international coalition of individuals, professionals and genetic support organizations that are working together to enhance the lives of everyone impacted by genetic conditions'. It goes on to say that it also includes, as part of its coalition of groups, 'public agencies, biotech companies, genetics diagnostic clinics, public health departments and children's hospitals, to name a few' (http://www. geneticalliance.org). That is, it seeks to bring together diverse public agencies and institutions, private organizations, and lay citizens in a broad alliance in pursuit of its goals. The Alliance sees its role as an educative one, aiming to inform the general public and providers about the personal and family ramifications of genetic testing, particularly through the publication of the first-hand experiences of members (Davidson *et al.*, 2000: 579). Such groups have a strong ethos of 'consumer' involvement and advocacy in research and policy decisions. For example, the Guiding Principles of the Genetic Alliance include phrases such as: 'Partnerships between consumers and professionals create powerful forces for change', and 'Meaningful progress in genetic research, policy and legislation requires consumer involvement' (http://www.geneticalliance.org/AboutUs/guidprinciples/html).

Members of support groups have actively lobbied for research in mapping genes, finding treatments, and discovering cures for particular genetic disorders. Their call for more research is in line with the view that genetic information provides the foundation for 'freedom of choice' and 'informed' decision-making. They often seek to forge links with private and public research organizations, with sympathetic professionals, and with biotech companies, and have sometimes played a crucial role in the setting of research priorities. In the US, for example, the Dystrophic Epidermolysis Bullosa Research Association of America has been successful in lobbying Congress for $5 million for research to cure this skin disease. Similarly, the Huntington Disease Society of America collected data that assisted in the eventual 'discovery' of the gene for Huntington's disease (Mackta and Weiss, 1994: 521). Such groups also seek to present consumer perspectives on the policy implications of genetic testing and the importance of consumer participation in the development of policy. The Genetic Alliance advocates the development of genetic testing protocols and informed-consent standards 'to ensure autonomous and informed decision-making that is founded on current, accurate information at every step of the testing, diagnostic and treatment-management process' (Davidson et al., 2000: 579).

The protection of consumer 'freedom of choice' and 'informed consent', and the promotion of public and professional 'genetic literacy', figure prominently as stated aims in accounts of these groups. The European Alliance of Genetic Support Groups (EAGS), founded in 1992, and representing 14 associations from 14 countries, draws heavily on the rhetoric of 'freedom of choice' and informed decision-making in its Statements and Guidelines (Poortman, 1999). Among other things, these note that: 'Needs-based *access to information* and facilities should be safeguarded'; and '*Individuals should be free to decide for themselves* whether or not to make use of the available information and facilities.' Furthermore, 'EAGS calls on behalf of families with genetic and congenital disorders for: *equal access to full information* ... [and] the *freedom of choice for all* within the legal framework of each country' (1999: 128; emphases added). Like other similar groups, the EAGS emphasizes the importance of research into the causes, prevention, diagnosis and treatment of genetic disorders and of public understanding of the need for such research. In the 'Commentary to the Statements and Guidelines', the benefits of genetic information for decision-making and the importance of voluntary action are repeatedly emphasized:

> *Knowing one's own and/or one's partner's genetic makeup creates options for action* regarding genetic testing and reproductive choice.... *There should be no third-party coercion.* This also applies to the option for prenatal diagnosis and *freedom to act upon the consequences.* Utilization of genetic services *must be voluntary.* Any pressure to utilize all available technology for diagnosis or risk assessment should be avoided.... *Genetic information can enable individuals to adopt strategies for reducing the risk of or preventing certain conditions*; e.g. lifestyle changes, dietary measures or the avoidance of certain occupational hazards.
>
> (Poortman, 1999: 129; emphases added)

During the 1992 meeting of EAGS in Copenhagen, problems ('bottlenecks') listed by the representatives of the various member organizations included lack of professional knowledge about genetics and lack of 'consumer' access and timely access to information. Identified priorities included increasing public awareness of genetics and genetic disorders, education of general practitioners, health authorities and teachers in matters relating to genetics, and the promotion of reproductive choice and screening (1999: 126–7).

Through their collaborative, educational, and lobbying efforts, genetic support groups and their umbrella organizations are an important 'vehicle' for forging or changing policies pertaining to new genetic technologies, and for advancing the ideals of active citizenship. Such groups have provided an important means of support to those affected by genetic disorders. However, because they tend to work in tandem with health professionals and scientists, and generally support their goals, it can be argued that they tend to buttress medical authority and corporate power. They offer no fundamental challenge to the genetic world view, which increasingly provides the foundation for social identity and social policies. The proliferation of these groups in recent years attests to the growing importance of categories of genetic risk and genetic disease to self-definition and group identity, and of the claim to 'freedom of choice' as a citizen right.

Other, more critical, views on genetics and 'freedom of choice'

Different, more critical perspectives have been offered by feminists, and members of disability rights groups and racial and ethnic minority rights groups. While also drawing heavily on the rhetoric of citizen rights and appealing to the value of 'informed decision-making', these critics tend to be sceptical about the extent of the 'freedoms' offered by new genetic technologies. In contrast to information technologies, which have highly problematic social and political implications but about which there has been a near-total absence of organized public concern, advances in biotechnology have become the focus of persistent public opposition (Nelkin, 1995). While there is no single critical standpoint with respect to new genetic technologies – there are differences of viewpoint both between *and* within the above groups – all share, to some extent, a concern about the potential for further social discrimination and exclusion arising from the routine use of new genetic technologies. While some groups, or subgroups, reject the new genetic technologies outright, others adopt a more cautious, qualified position, drawing attention to the dangers of the unreflective and unregulated use of genetic technologies. The social priority, it is argued, should be changing those social arrangements that predispose to sexism, homophobia, racism, ethnocentrism, and disablism, and that constrain 'choice', rather than the expansion of access to new genetic technologies. Mindful of past eugenic and biomedical abuses, commentators have drawn attention to the potential for genetic selection. They have underlined the ways in which genetic technologies may be used to extend control over bodies and lives by imposing or 'fixing' identities, excluding categories of 'the undesirable' and creating imperatives that *limit* options. The groups have engaged to varying degrees in a vigorous public debate about the implications of the new genetic technologies, and seek to promote their views through scholarly publications, the media, and other public forums. Here we focus on the arguments of feminists and disability rights groups, who have contributed substantially to debates on the impacts of new genetic technologies in recent years. (For an overview of minority group, particularly racial and ethnic minority group, responses, see Zilinskas and Balint, 2001 and Mittman *et al.*, 1998.)

Feminist perspectives

There is a large and theoretically diverse body of feminist scholarship that critically examines the notion of 'freedom of choice' in relation to new reproductive technologies in general, and genetic-based prenatal testing and genetic counselling in particular. Although virtually all versions of feminism accept 'self-determination' as a basic premise, the issue of choice – what it means for women who decide to use reproductive technologies, and those unable to exercise it at all – is hotly contested (Petersen, 1994: 29). A common view, expressed by Spallone and Steinberg, is that choices made between limited, undesirable or negative alternatives hardly amount to choices at all (1987: 29). For example, one needs to question what choice means in reproductive decision-making in a society which puts a high priority on motherhood, which is seen as central to women's definition, and where options are limited by women's class, 'race', age, marital status, sexual preference, religion, culture and disability. Notions of 'normal' parenthood and the 'fit' mother, which tend to exclude women who are single, lesbian, disabled or older, are seen to provide a powerful constraint on 'freedom of choice' (Spallone and Steinberg, 1987: 7–8).

Under the influence of recent theoretical trends such as postmodernism/poststructuralism, anti-racist/black theory, and queer theory, and a shift away from an exclusive focus on gender, feminists have increasingly given recognition to the multiple constraints on 'choice' offered by factors such as 'race', sexuality, class, and disability. For example, in her study of in vitro fertilization and genetic screening, Steinberg explores how IVF technologies and screening practices reflect and reinforce different social divisions, particularly through the language of genetic risks, which allows the profiling of offspring and 'genetified selections' (1997: 95–100). As Steinberg argues, voluntary action and 'freedom of choice' in reproductive decisions is problematic in a context of medically defined risk:

The call for voluntary screening places putative emphasis on patients' choice and on the perception that genetic counselling and screening enable patients to make difficult decisions. Yet, it is questionable what 'choice' might mean in the context of the language of 'risk'. In this context, a practitioner's willingness to proceed 'if couples accept the risks' underestimates the power of negative medical discourses of disability, and medical judgements expressed in the ableist language of 'risk'. Considering the ableism endemic in our social institutions and dominant social (including medical) attitudes, how many patients would be willing to proceed with treatment if advised that there was 'risk' of producing disabled offspring?

(1997: 98)

Many feminists have identified biomedicine as a major source of constraint on 'choice' in relation to reproductive decision-making. As has been argued, biomedical ideologies and practices powerfully shape issues and lives; for example, prenatal testing shapes the experiences and progression of pregnancy, views on abortion, attitudes to disability, and perspectives on ageing (Lippman, 1992: 148–50). Despite this, biomedicine tends to exclude women's interests and perspectives. The use of gender-neutral language in reproductive genetics – as in references to 'parental rights and responsibilities' – denies that it is women's bodies that undergo discomfort and risk in the course of prenatal testing (Mahowald, 1994: 69). As Abby Lippman (1992) explains, prenatal testing is presented in biomedical narratives as an activity to reduce the frequency of selective birth defects, as a way of enhancing 'reproductive autonomy'. Although it might give women some control over their pregnancies, respecting their autonomy to choose the kinds of children they will bear, it is also an assembly-line approach to the products of conception, which allows the separation of the 'desirable' and 'undesirable' 'products'. Women may seem to choose, but their only options are those already created by biomedicine. For example, continuing a pregnancy when the foetus has been found to have Down syndrome is not a realistic alternative in a society that does not accept children with disabilities (1992: 144–7). On the basis of such observations, some feminists conclude that reproductive medicine is invested in, and formative of, eugenic ideologies of family and breeding (e.g. Steinberg, 1997: 75–8).

Feminists differ on the question of whether or not new genetic-based reproductive technologies should be rejected outright. Some groups, such as the Feminist International Network on Resistance to Reproductive and Genetic Engineering (FINRRAGE), are opposed to the new technologies on the grounds of the physical, psychological and political risks they pose to women. However, others, particularly those who have been influenced by the recent 'poststructural' turn in social theory, recognize the productive power of new genetic technologies, and the potential they create for social identity and social action, including contestation. In the view of Sawicki (1991), for example, the new reproductive technologies are not simply tools of patriarchal domination, but rather constitute 'disciplinary technologies' that generate new categories of individual (e.g. the infertile, surrogate and genetically impaired mothers, mothers whose bodies are not fit for pregnancy, etc.) and potential new sites of resistance. As Sawicki argues, it is important to recognize that part of the attraction of the new reproductive technologies is that *many women perceive them as enabling*, as offering new identities and specific kinds of solutions to the dilemmas they face (1991: 85). Sawicki contends that 'analyses that simply reject new reproductive technologies do not assist women in making choices' (1991: 92). Rather than simply reject the technologies outright on the grounds that they do violence to women's bodies, one should create space for women who are affected by the technologies to voice their views on their needs, and their experiences of pregnancy and childbirth. Women should be given the opportunity to assess the risks and benefits, and have access to those technologies which they deem beneficial (1991: 89–92).

One of the primary goals of recent feminist work in relation to new genetic-based reproductive technologies has indeed been to 'give voice' to women's experiences, by wresting control of definitions from the experts. In Rayna Rapp's (1999) recent exploration of the social impact and cultural meaning of prenatal diagnosis – 'one of the most routinized of the new reproductive technologies' – an effort is made to deconstruct the language of choice and give expression to the experiences of women from diverse backgrounds. In her ethnographic 'women-centred analysis', she reveals the tensions that exist between the scientific definitions of risk, heredity, and control expounded by genetic counsellors and other experts, and the popular conceptions of the same domain that women and their supporters from diverse backgrounds express.

Counsellors' chromosomal explanation of disability was often found to conflict with some patients' causal explanations, which may invoke, say, migration or life experiences, a troubled family medical history, birth order, or religious intervention (Rapp, 1999: 82–93). As Rapp's work shows, women are by no means powerless in their relationships with counsellors, geneticists, and other experts. Despite constraints on 'choice', imposed by the routinization of prenatal care for some sectors of the population, 'there are those who choose not to accept its complicated benefits and burdens' (1999: 167). Women's prior knowledge about the test, gleaned from books, friends, and private physicians, 'practical sense of community epidemiology', religious beliefs, and fear of miscarriage are among some of the factors likely to influence the decision to refuse a test (1999: 165–90).

In her analysis of Sickle Cell Disease (SCD) in low-income families, Shirley Hill (1994) has sought to 'give voice' to black mothers who are involved in the day-to-day medical and home care of children with SCD. Specifically, she is concerned with caregiving in the context of non-traditional families, highlighting the roles of 'race', class, culture, and gender in women's perceptions and responses to illness and caregiving options. Hill notes that family diversity has been largely ignored in family caregiving studies. Even with the shift in medical care from hospitals to families, recent studies 'still view the family as a nuclear entity formed by marriage' (1994: 7). Like Rapp, Hill shows that women make complex responses to medical intervention, shaped by 'a history of doubting medical authority and regimes', previous personal experience with professionals, and values surrounding motherhood. Women's responses were found to be often at odds with the medical response, which focuses on the 'objective, scientific' facts: the etiology and transmission of the disease, statistical risk assessment, treatment and prognosis of the affected, and the elimination of SCD by early detection of the trait and selective reproduction. Genetic screening had minimal effect on reproductive behaviour, in part because women received inadequate medical information about the disease, but also because women valued their ability to have children. Women showed little interest in medical explanations of causation and genetic transmission of the disease, had difficulty tracing the sickle cell trait in their families, and sometimes doubted that their children really had the disease. Hill shows how the women achieved greater control over managing SCD by *rejecting* the medical model of the disease. Mothers emphasized their children's normality rather than their illness, and 'were often more tolerant of illness symptoms than health professionals were, which helped them minimize the impact of the disease on their children'. Despite social constraints, women were able to express their agency in coping with SCD in diverse ways: by redefining unmanageable aspects of SCD in manageable ways, obfuscating the reproductive implications of carrying the trait, and using 'stress-reducing normalization and denial as coping strategies' (1994: 8–9).

Disability rights perspectives

In the same way that feminists have sought to 'give voice' to women's views, disability scholars and activists have argued for fairer representation of the views of disabled people in public debates and policies. Women's right to choose is generally supported, but the context in which choice is exercised is deplored. While there are similarities between the perspective of 'second-wave' feminism and the social model of disability (particularly the privileging of experience), indeed feminism has been used as a point of comparison and as a tool to constructively critique the latter, one needs to be cautious when comparing perspectives. As with the category 'women', there has been a tendency to view 'disabled people' as comprising an undifferentiated unitary grouping, and to overlook differences in experience and perspective according to gender, age, 'race', ethnicity, and impairment (Fawcett, 2000: 5–6). However, as with feminisms, the concern about 'freedom of choice' and its meanings is a point of commonality among diverse disability groups. As some writers observe, there is a tension between the goals of enhancing reproductive choice (the position supported by many feminists) and preventing the births of children who would have disabilities (a policy that is generally resisted by disability rights scholars and activists). A final draft position statement of the British Council of Disabled People (BCODP) notes that:

> There can be no informed choice as long as genetic counselling is directive and continues to misinform women about the experience of disability. There can be no free choice as long as prejudice against and fear of disabled people continues. There can be no real choice until women feel able to continue with a pregnancy, secure in the knowledge that they will be bringing a

child into a society which positively welcomes all children and provides comprehensive systems of support.

(BCODP, undated)

Disability scholars and activists argue that disability has been medicalized, and there has been a tendency to focus on the impairment almost to the exclusion of the person. There has been a lack of critical examination of the social context within which the technologies are developed, and a devaluing of the lives of those who already have disabilities (Bailey, 1996: 144). Because they tend to live longer than men and are subject to a disproportionate burden of poverty, disabled women, it has been argued, are especially vulnerable to genetic discrimination (Kallianes and Rubenfeld, 1997; Rock, 1996). In genetic counselling, information is limited to the provision of data on genetic risk, while information about disability in contemporary society and what it means to bring up a disabled child is lacking. Disability scholars' and activists' concerns about discrimination arising from the use of new genetic technologies would seem to be well founded. A thirty-six nation survey on 'patients' and professionals' views on autonomy, disability and "discrimination"', conducted between 1993 and 1995, revealed that patients, geneticists and primary care physicians tend to share a pessimistic view of disability. It was found that most thought that some disabilities would never be overcome, and that society would never provide enough services. Few believed that people with severe disabilities added to society (Wertz, 1999: 174).

The resurgence of eugenics is of particular concern to many people with disabilities, in light of increasing pressure on women (particularly disabled women) to undergo prenatal genetic testing, and the presumption that having a positive test result will inevitably be followed by an abortion (see, for example, Hume, 1996; Shakespeare, 1998). Eugenics via non-coercive individual choices, what Tom Shakespeare calls 'weak eugenics' (1998: 669), is seen as a strong possibility in the current context of cost cutting, through a reduction in expenditure for health and welfare, including the care of the chronically ill. According to Bailey (1996), the reluctance of the state to intervene to limit the use of genetic technology which is seen to encroach on the rights of individual choice, and a growing emphasis on cost-benefit analysis and consumerism in health care, combine to create pressures to selectively abort. She notes: 'There would seem to be a precariously thin line dividing the aim of preventing impairment in the interests of society, which could be eugenic in effect if not intent, from the aims of enabling women to make an informed choice' (1996: 162). Consequently, greater attention needs to be given to the ways in which choices are constrained both by social circumstances and by the experience of testing itself (1996: 164).

As Adrienne Asch (1989) observes, advocates of disability rights and feminists share important beliefs and values in their affirmation of the right to 'self-determination' (1989: 107). Thus, one can support a pro-choice perspective, but challenge the view of disability that lies behind the endorsement of genetic testing and the assumption that women should end their pregnancies if they discover that the foetus has a disabling trait (Asch, 1999). Like feminists, disability scholars and activists are critical of the medicalization of problems, and draw attention to the constraints on 'choice' offered by medical ideologies and technological options. Asch observes that while the medical and public health establishment endorses efforts to improve the lives of existing human beings through improvements in environment and lifestyle, and provides prenatal care to pregnant women, it fails to see that the future disabled child is more than just an impairment (1999: 1651–2). She is especially concerned with the perspective on life with disability that is communicated by the effort to develop prenatal testing, facilitated in particular by new genetic technologies, and urge it on every pregnant woman. While prenatal screening and diagnosis may be beneficial for individual women and families, the proliferation of such technologies contributes to the medicalization of pregnancy and creates pressures to abort after diagnoses of disability (Asch, 1989: 82–3). Disability scholars emphasize that the definitions of terms such as 'health', 'normality' and 'disability' are not objective and universal across time and place. Rather, they are evaluated within a society at a particular time according to shared perceptions of what is typical functioning and what are typical roles for people. The dominance of the medically oriented understanding of disabilities has tended to focus attention on the continuous disruption in the life of the disabled person and to view all problems that occur to people with disabilities as attributable to the condition itself rather than to external factors. If disability is viewed in social, minority-group terms, however, one would see that rules, laws, timetables, buildings, transport systems, etc., exclude some people from full participation in social life (Asch, 1999: 1650–1).

Like early feminist writers who distinguished between sex (biological difference of male and female) and gender (the social experience of being a man or woman), disabled people distinguish impairment (a bodily difference) from disability (society's treatment of people with impairments) (Shakespeare and Erickson, 2000: 194). In their view, the problem is not the impairment per se, but society's response to the impairment ('being disabled'). As Shakespeare explains: 'Impairment is not the defining characteristic of being a disabled person, because everyone experiences degrees of illness and impairment' (Shakespeare, 1998: 671). According to many writers, the presumption that most people who attend prenatal counselling sessions will choose to undergo testing needs to be challenged. In Germany and the Netherlands, at least, the response of organizations representing disabled people to genetic counselling has been to claim a 'right to abnormality', the argument being that the resulting diversity can strengthen a community (Hepburn, 1998: 39). However, as Asch argues, if there is 'an unshakable commitment to the technology in the name of reproductive choice', practitioners should change their practices, including the way information about impairments detected in the foetus is delivered (Asch, 1999: 1655). For example, genetic counsellors should seek to understand what parents desire in childrearing and how a disabling condition in general or a specific type of impairment would affect their hopes and expectations of parenthood (1999: 1655; see also Asch, 1989: 90–92; Parens and Asch, 1999).

In summary, feminists and disability scholars and activists share many concerns about new genetic technologies and are critical of the notion that the technologies will necessarily promote autonomy or 'freedom of choice'. Commentators have drawn attention to the ways in which these technologies may constrain freedom, particularly by establishing new imperatives in relation to reproduction, such as the imperative to abort and to perfect human beings. They have interrogated the meaning of choice, especially in light of the prevalent consumerist ethos in health care, and the retreat of the state from regulation over new genetic technologies. Constraints are diverse and, as feminists indicate, are likely to have a different impact on different categories of people, defined by the interplay of gender, class, 'race', ethnicity, sexuality, dis/ability, and so on. Feminists and disability scholars and activists have critiqued biological determinism – the notion that 'it's all in the genes' – and express similar fears about eugenic outcomes, resulting from the operations of 'the market'. However, few writers from these or other areas of critical scholarship take issue with the ideal of 'self-determination' or the potential for individuals to act in a relatively unconstrained way given the 'right' conditions. Indeed, some, such as Rapp and Hill, have sought to show that people are, at least to some extent, able to negotiate, subvert, and contest the norms and imperatives with which they are confronted. Biomedical authority and regimes may represent a dominating influence on our lives, but people are not powerless and there is always scope for 'non-normative' or alternative courses of action. In light of the above and the foregoing chapters, we wish to draw some conclusions on active citizenship and new genetic technologies, and suggest some further avenues for exploration and action.

Some conclusions on active citizenship and new genetic technologies, and suggestions for further exploration and action

As we have argued, active citizenship is a pervasive discourse in many contemporary societies, providing the framework for many discussions about new genetic technologies and their purported benefits, as well as the rationale for diverse programmes and practices. Both proponents and critics of new genetic technologies draw on the concept and use the language of active citizenship in debates. However, as noted above, there are contending views on the question of what active citizenship means, or might mean, in practice. The widespread appeal of the ideal of active citizenship, combined with lack of agreement on how it should be realized, means that it is open to easy appropriation by different authorities and constituencies for their own particular purposes. The claim of critical scholars that individuals have a 'right' to be 'self-determining', for instance, is not inconsistent with the neo-liberal view that individuals should 'stand on their own feet', by relying less on the state for support and making provision for their own current welfare and future well-being. In a neo-liberal context, characterized by the pervasive values of consumerism and individualism, there is a danger that those who use the language of active citizenship may unwittingly reinforce the trend described by Miringoff (1991), namely the increasing replacement of social welfare by genetic welfare. (See Chapter 2.) Consumerism embodies the notion of the essentially autonomous, rational, 'selfish' individual, who is 'driven' primarily by expectations of pleasure and gain (material benefits and 'choices') derived from participation in 'the market'. In contemporary societies, consumption is central to constructions of 'self' and 'other', and to delineating boundaries of 'social identity', as group membership or identification, and is therefore inherently exclusionary (Falk, 1994: 133–8). It is important to recognize that consumption has become institutionalized not as a right or pleasure, but as the *duty* of the citizen (Baudrillard, 1998: 80), and that 'the market' is implicated in the generation of many social divisions and inequalities.

In a 'free market' economy not everyone is able to 'participate' equally in decision-making about the introduction of new genetic technologies, and not everyone has access to the conditions, products, and services that are seen as necessary to maintaining or advancing health and wellbeing. The increasingly deregulated, globalized market that fuels, and is fuelled by, rampant consumerism indeed arguably contributes to many of the diseases that new genetic technologies are expected to redress. A significant proportion of cancers and chronic illness conditions have been attributed to the workings of the unregulated market: lack of access to meaningful, well-paid employment, poor working conditions, inadequate provision of housing, over-consumption of resources, a polluted environment, and so on. In efforts to realize active citizenship, it is important not to lose sight of the kinds of large-scale structural changes that need to be made, and the kinds of social alliances that need to be forged, in order to reduce inequalities in standards of living and health. With the redefinition of concepts of self and society accompanying the genetic world view, and the extension of free-market thinking and consumerism to more and more domains of life, there is a need to critically evaluate political responses and strategies, and such basic concepts as 'oppression', 'constraint', 'rights', 'freedom', and 'choice'. Developments in new genetic technologies offer both opportunities and dangers for individuals and groups. It is important that both proponents and critics of these technologies reflect upon their use of terminology and categories, and recognize how they shape and may limit what can be known about the impact of the technologies on people's lives and relationships.

The implications of adopting the language and assumptions of 'the new genetics', we contend, need to be thoroughly explored, particularly in light of the generally positive media 'framing' of genetics and its benefits, described in Chapter 4. Very often the terminology and perspectives of genetics are taken up and used by writers in an unreflective way, without recognizing how they convey particular views of body, self and society. As mentioned in Chapter 2, in recent writings the term 'new genetics' itself is often left undefined, while the 'new genetics'/old eugenics dichotomy remains unquestioned. Further, as noted in Chapter 5, despite trenchant criticisms of genetic counsellors' language and preferred approach ('non-directiveness'), offered by counsellors themselves and others, assumptions about client autonomy and the neutrality of genetic information continue to inform professional practice. Recent work in the social sciences and humanities has highlighted the ways in which language constitutes our reality, and how terms and categories may serve to limit thought, define paths of action, and regulate lives and relationships. The ideals of 'freedom of choice' and 'participation' have, without doubt, proved valuable to many social movements (e.g. civil rights, feminist, gay and lesbian rights, disability rights) in past struggles. However, the limitations of the so-called 'identity politics' upon which these movements have relied, and continue largely to rely, have become increasingly evident in recent years (Petersen, 1998b: 12–14). Within the framework of 'identity politics', 'freedom' tends to be conceived as the absence of constraint on 'the true self' and on action, as though there were some ideal state of unconstraint outside social relations. This idealistic conception of freedom has limited possibilities for social action and social change. As one writer comments: 'Freedom does not basically lie in discovering or being able to determine who we are, but in rebelling against those ways in which we are already defined, categorized, and classified' (Rajchman, 1984, cited by Sawicki, 1991: 27). In the same way that feminists and gay and lesbian scholars have in the past highlighted how biomedical categories such as the hysterical woman and the homosexual have oppressed women and gays, respectively, there is a need to expose how genetic categories define and limit ways of being. The terms 'the genetically diseased' and the 'genetically at risk' are not simply descriptive terms – which designate an already existing objective condition or state of being – but have constitutive power and evaluative connotations. They create identity labels and suggest preferred forms of response.

Having said this, it is important to acknowledge and accept that, at the level of the individual, people are likely to have mixed views on new genetic technologies and have complex reactions to genetic language and information. Some people may believe that they are 'empowered' by new genetic offerings, and may wish 'to know' about their genetic makeup and identify themselves by genetic terms. Their 'reasons' for these beliefs and desires are also likely to be complex and need to be acknowledged, although one might query in what sense they believe they are 'empowered', or what it is exactly they wish 'to know'. Also, people who are affected by genetic disorders, or who have been diagnosed as being 'at risk' of a genetic disorder, may be critical of biomedical language and labels, but still personally value knowledge about their disorders and wish to actively participate in their treatment. (See, for example, Mary Ann Beall's (1996) account, where she criticizes medical labelling but acknowledges the importance of genetic information in her own recovery from and coping with mental illness.) On the other hand, others may experience new genetic technologies as threatening, may not want to be informed about their genetic risk or 'know' whether their condition has a genetic basis, and may eschew genetic labels. Contributors to the recent ethical debate about people's 'right to know' or 'right not to know' acknowledge these complexities. They recognize that the provision of genetic information, which in the event only deals with probabilities, may be experienced as either 'empowering' or serve to undermine 'autonomy' and 'self-determination' and threaten an individual's integrity or 'sense of self' (Chadwick, 1997: 19–20). In this book, we have not offered conclusions on how people *should* respond to the new genetic technologies – whether they should be embraced or rejected – and have not explored in any detail how they *have* responded thus far. Rather, we have sought to identify some of the governing discourses surrounding 'the new genetics' as they are seen to affect the health of 'the public' and some emergent developments that are likely to profoundly affect a significant number of people. Our aim has been to stimulate further debate and research on this topic, with the hope that the new imperative to 'know thyself' in genetic terms does not preclude critical reflection.

Bibliography

Adam, B. (2000) 'The temporal gaze: the challenge for social theory in the context of GM food', *British Journal of Sociology*, 51, 3: 125–42.

Allan, S., Adam, B. and Carter, C. (2000) *Environmental Risks and the Media*, London and New York: Routledge.

Allen, G. (1996) 'Science misapplied: the eugenic age revisited', *Technology Review*, August/September: 23–31.

Allen, G. (1999) 'Modern biological determinism: the Violence Initiative, the Human Genome Project, and the New Eugenics', in M. Fortun and E. Mendelsohn (eds) *The Practices of Human Genetics*, Dordrecht: Kluwer Academic Publishers.

Amalfi, C. (1999a) 'Genetic jigsaw falls neatly into place', *The West Australian*, 5 April: 17.

Amalfi, C. (1999b) 'Mad scientist image distorts clone debate', *The West Australian*, 18 March: 8.

Anderson, W. T. (2000) 'The two globalizations: notes on a confused dialogue', *Futures*, 31: 9–10.

Andrews, L. B. (1996) 'Prenatal screening and the culture of motherhood', *Hastings Law Journal*, 47, 4: 967–1006.

Appleyard, B. (1998) *Brave New Worlds: Staying Human in the Genetic Future*, New York: Viking.

Armour, A. (1995) 'The citizens' jury model of public participation: a critical evaluation', in O. Renn, T. Webler and P. Wiedmann (eds) *Fairness and Competence in Citizen Participation: Evaluating Models of Environmental Discourse*, Dordrecht: Kluwer Academic Publishers.

Armstrong, D. (1993) 'Public health spaces and the fabrication of identity', *Sociology*, 27, 3: 393–410.

Armstrong, D. (1995) 'The rise of surveillance medicine', *The Sociology of Health and Illness*, 17: 393–404.

Armstrong, D., Michie, S. and Marteau, T. (1998) 'Revealed identity: a study of the process of genetic counselling', *Social Science and Medicine*, 47, 11: 1653–8.

Asch, A. (1989) 'Reproductive technology and disability', in S. Cohen and N. Taub (eds) *Reproductive Laws for the 1990s*, Clifton, NJ: Humana Press.

Asch, A. (1999) 'Prenatal diagnosis and selective abortion: a challenge to practice and policy', *American Journal of Public Health*, 89, 11: 1649–57.

Ashton, J. (ed) (1992) *Healthy Cities*, Milton Keynes: Open University Press.

Ashton, J. and Seymour, H. (1988) *The New Public Health*, Milton Keynes: Open University Press.

Atkinson, P., Batchelor, C. and Parsons, E. (1997) 'The rhetoric of prediction and chance in the research to clone a disease gene', in M. A. Elston (ed.) *The Sociology of Medical Science and Technology*, Oxford: Blackwell.

Austin, M. A. and Peyser, P. A. (2000) 'The multidisciplinary nature of public health genetics in research and education', in M. J. Khoury, W. Burke and E. J. Thomson (eds) *Genetics and Public Health in the 21st Century: Using Genetic Information to Improve Health and Prevent Disease*, New York: Oxford University Press.

Baggott, R. (2000) *Public Health Policy and Politics*, New York: St Martin's Press.

Bailey, P. (2001) 'The people's science: involving consumers in scientific research', *Wellcome News*, 26: 6–7.

Bailey, R. (1996) 'Prenatal testing and the prevention of impairment: a woman's right to choose?', in J. Morris (ed.) *Encounters with Strangers: Feminism and Disability*, London: The Women's Press Ltd.

Bainbridge, J., Ellahi, B., Smith, G. and Whisson, J. (eds) (2000) *Genetically Modified Foods: A Practical Guide for Business*, Oxford: Chandos.

Baker, C. (undated) *Your Genes, Your Choices: Exploring the Issues Raised by Genetic Research*, American Association for the Advancement of Science.

Bartley, M., Davey-Smith, C. and Blane, D. (1997) 'Vital comparisons: the social construction of mortality measurement', in M. A. Elston (ed.) *The Sociology of Medical Science and Technology*, Oxford: Blackwell.

Baudrillard, J. (1998) *The Consumer Society: Myths and Structures*, London: Sage.

Bauman, Z. (1997) *Postmodernity and its Discontents*, Cambridge: Polity Press.

Beale, B. (1997) 'Forget the Elvis scenarios, it's time for sensible debate', *The Sydney Morning Herald*, 25 February: 8.

Beall, M. A. (1996) 'A hunger for knowledge and respect', in L. L. Hall (ed.) *Genetics and Mental Illness: Evolving Issues for Research and Society*, New York and London: Plenum Press.

Beck, U. (1992) *Risk Society*, London: Sage.

Beck, U. (2000) 'The cosmopolitan perspective: sociology of the second age of modernity', *British Journal of Sociology*, 51, 1: 79–105.

Beck-Gernsheim, E. (1995) *The Social Implications of Bioengineering*, Atlantic Highlands, NJ: Humanities Press.

Beck-Gernsheim, E. (1996) 'Life as a planning project', in S. Lash, B. Szerszynski and D. Wynne (eds) *Risk, Environment and Modernity: Towards a New Ecology*, London: Sage.

Bell, J. (1998) 'The new genetics and clinical practice', *British Medical Journal*, 316, 7131: 618–20.

Benedick, R. E. (1999) 'Tomorrow's environment is global', *Futures*, 31, 9–10: 937–47.

Berg, M. (1997) *Rationalizing Medical Work: Decision-Support Techniques and Medical Practice*, Cambridge, MA: MIT Press.

Biesecker, B. B. (1997) 'Privacy in genetic counselling', in M. A. Rothstein (ed.) *Genetic Secrets: Protecting Privacy and Confidentiality in the Genetic Era*, New Haven and London: Yale University Press.

Binyon, M. (1999) 'Prognosis of a whole country', *The Australian*, 24 February: 39.

Birkett, D. (2000) 'Are you a good citizen?', *The Guardian*, 12 December: 5.

Bloom, F. E. (1997) 'Editorial: breakthroughs 1997', *Science*, 19 December, 278: 2029.

Bogard, W. (1996) *The Simulation of Surveillance: Hypercontrol in Telematic Societies*, Cambridge: Cambridge University Press.

Bosk, C. L. (1992) *All God's Mistakes: Genetic Counseling in a Pediatric Hospital*, Chicago and London: The University of Chicago Press.

Boulyjenkov, V. (1998) 'WHO Human Genetics Programme: a brief overview', *Community Genetics*, 1: 57–60.

Bower, A. (1997) 'Brain disorder genes offer hope', *The West Australian*, 13 September: 54.

Brandt-Rauf, P. W. and Brandt-Rauf, S. I. (1997) 'Biomarkers: scientific advances and societal implications', in M. A. Rothstein (ed.) *Genetic Secrets: Protecting Privacy and Confidentiality in the Genetic Era*, New Haven and London: Yale University Press.

British Council of Disabled People (undated) 'Final draft BCODP position statement and list of demands on disability and the new genetics' [publisher not known].

British Medical Association (1998) *Human Genetics: Choice and Responsibility*, Oxford and New York: Oxford University Press.

Brock, S. C. (1995) 'Narrative and medical genetics: on ethics and therapeutics', *Qualitative Health Research*, 5, 2: 150–68.

Brook, S. (2001) 'Gene discovery may alleviate obesity, diabetes', *The Weekend Australian*, 10–11 February: 15.

Brookbank, C. (1999) 'Disease models: relevance is everything', *Molecular Medicine Today*, 5: 274.

Brundtland Report, The (1987) *Our Common Future*, Oxford: Oxford University Press, World Commission on Environment and Development.

Brunger, F. and Lippman, A. (1995) 'Resistance and adherence to the norms of genetic counseling', *Journal of Genetic Counseling*, 4, 3: 151–67.

Buchanan, A., Brock, D. W., Daniels, N. and Wikler, D. (2000) *From Chance to Choice: Genetics and Justice*, Cambridge: Cambridge University Press.

Buckley, J.J. (1978) *Genetics Now: Ethical Issues in Genetic Research*, Washington: University Press of America.

Bunton, R. (2001) 'Knowledge, embodiment and neo-liberal drug policy', *Contemporary Drug Problems*, Summer: 221–43.

Bunton, R., Nettleton, S. and Burrows, R. (eds) (1995) *The Sociology of Health Promotion: Critical Analyses of Consumption, Lifestyle and Risk*, London and New York: Routledge.

Burchell, G., Gordon, C. and Miller, P. (eds) (1991) *The Foucault Effect: Studies in Governmentality*, London: Harvester Wheatsheaf.

Burke, D. (2000) 'The recent excitement over genetically modified foods', in B. Adam, U. Beck and J. Van Loon (eds) *Risk Society and Beyond: Critical Issues for Social Theory*, London: Sage.

Burrows, R. and Pleace, N. (eds) (2000) *Wired Welfare, Discussion Document*, York: University of York, Centre for Housing Studies.

Butler, D. and Wadman, M. (1997) 'Calls for cloning ban sell science short', *Nature*, 386, 6620: 8–9.

Buttel, F. (1999) 'Agricultural biotechnology: its recent evolution and implications for agrifood political economy', *Sociological Research Online*, 4, 3.

Callaghan, G. (1996) 'Gene genie', *The Weekend Australian*, 14 December: 2.

Capecchi, M. R. (2000) 'Human germline gene therapy', in G. Stock and J. Campbell (eds) *Engineering the Human Germline: An Exploration of the Science and Ethics of Altering the Genes We Pass to Our Children*, New York and Oxford: Oxford University Press.

Cartwright, A. (1967) *Patients and their Doctors*, London and New York: Routledge and Kegan Paul.

Cassel, C. K. (1997) 'Policy implications of the Human Genome Project for women', *Women's Health Issues*, 7, 4: 225–9.

Castel, R. (1981) *La Gestion des risques, de l'anti-psychiatrie à l'après-psychanalyse*, Paris: Minuit.

Castells, M. (1996) *The Rise of Network Society*, Oxford: Blackwell.

Chadwick, R. (1993) 'What counts as success in genetic counselling?', *Journal of Medical Ethics*, 19: 43–6.

Chadwick, R. (1997) 'The philosophy of the right to know and the right not to know', in R. Chadwick, M. Levitt and D. Shickle (eds) *The Right to Know and the Right not to Know*, Aldershot: Ashgate.

Chadwick, R. and Levitt, M. (1996) 'Euroscreen: ethical and philosophical issues of genetic screening in Europe', *Journal of the Royal College of Physicians of London*, 30, 1: 67–9.

Chadwick, R., Levitt, M. and Shickle, D. (eds) (1997) *The Right to Know and the Right Not to Know*, Aldershot: Ashgate.

Chapple, A., May, C. and Campion, P. (1995) 'Lay understanding of genetic disease: a British study of families attending a genetic counseling service', *Journal of Genetic Counseling*, 4, 4: 281–300.

Check, W. A. (1995) 'Genetic counselling: your new job', *ACP-ASIM Observer*, February: 1–10 (http://www.acponline.org/journals/news/feb95/gencoun.htm).

Chu, C. (1994) 'Integrating health and environment: the key to an ecological public health', in C. Chu and R. Simpson (eds) *Ecological Public Health: From Vision to Practice*, Canada and Aus. Inst. of Applied Environ. Research Griffith University and Centre for Health Promotion Toronto Canada.

Chynoweth, C. (1998) 'Genes clue to relief', *The Weekend Australian*, 16–17 May: 41.

Clague, J. (1998) 'Genetic knowledge as a commodity: the Human Genome Project, markets and consumers', in M. Junker-Kenny and L. S. Cahill (eds), *The Ethics of Genetic Engineering*, London: SCM Press and Maryknoll, NY: Orbis Books.

Clarke, A. (1990) 'Genetics, ethics and audit', *The Lancet*, 335: 1145–7.

Clarke, A. (1991) 'Is non-directive counselling possible?', *The Lancet*, 338: 998–1001.

Clarke, A. (1997a) 'The process of genetic counselling: beyond non-directiveness', in P. S. Harper and A. J. Clarke (eds) *Genetics, Society and Clinical Practice*, Oxford: Bios Scientific Publishers.

Clarke, A. (1997b) 'Outcomes and process in genetic counselling', in P. S. Harper and A. J. Clarke (eds) *Genetics, Society and Clinical Practice*, Oxford: Bios Scientific Publishers.

Clarke, A., Parsons, E. and Williams, A. (1996) 'Outcomes and process in genetic counselling', *Clinical Genetics*, 50: 462–9.

Coburn D. (2000) 'Income inequality, social cohesion and the health status of populations: the role of neo-liberalism', *Social Science and Medicine*, 51: 135–46.

Cohen, M. J. (1997) 'Risk society and ecological modernisation: alternative visions for post-industrial nations', *Futures*, 29, 2: 105–19.

Conrad, P. (1997) 'Public eyes and private genes: historical frames, news constructions, and social problems', *Social Problems*, 44, 2: 139–54.

Conrad, P. (1999) 'Uses of expertise: sources, quotes, and voice in the reporting of genetics in the news', *Public Understanding of Science*, 8: 285–302.

Conrad, P. (2001) 'Genetic optimism: framing genes and mental illness in the news', *Culture, Medicine and Psychiatry*, 25: 225–47.

Conrad, P. and Gabe, J. (1999a) *Sociological Perspectives on the New Genetics*, Oxford: Blackwell.

Conrad, P. and Gabe, J. (1999b) 'Introduction: Sociological perspectives on the new genetics: an overview', *Sociology of Health and Illness*, 21, 5: 505–16.

Coote, A. and Lenaghan, J. (1997) *Citizens' Juries: Theory into Practice*, London: Institute for Public Policy Research.

Cranor, C. F. (1994) 'Genetic causation', in C. F. Cranor (ed.) *Are Genes Us? The Social Consequences of the New Genetics*, New Brunswick, NJ: Rutgers University Press.

Cronberg, T. (1995) 'Do marginal voices shape technology?', in S. Joss and J. Durant (eds) *Public Participation in Science: The Role of Consensus Conferences in Europe*, London: Science Museum.

Crossley, M. A. (1996) 'Choice, conscience, and context', *Hastings Law Journal*, 47, 4: 1223–39.

Cunningham-Burley, S. and Kerr, A. (1999) 'Defining the "social": towards an understanding of scientific and medical discourses on the social aspects of the new human genetics', *Sociology of Health and Illness*, 21, 5: 647–68.

Cuomo, C. J. (1998) *Feminism and Ecological Communities: An Ethic of Flourishing*, London and New York: Routledge.

Dale, P. J. (1999) 'Public reactions and scientific responses to transgenic crops', *Current Opinion in Biotechnology*, 10, 2: 203–8.

Daniel, A. (1998) 'Trust and medical authority', in A. Petersen and C. Waddell (eds) *Health Matters: A Sociology of Illness, Prevention and Care*, Sydney: Allen & Unwin.

Darnovsky, M. (2001) 'The new eugenics: the case against genetically modified humans', in B. Tokar (ed.), *Redesigning Life? The Worldwide Challenge to Genetic Engineering*, New York: Zed Books.

Davidson, M. E., David, K., Hsu, N., Pollin, T. I., Weiss, J. O., Wilker, N. and Wilson, M. A. (2000) 'Consumer perspectives on genetic testing: lessons learned', in M. J. Khoury, W. Burke and E. J. Thomson (eds) *Genetics and Public Health in the 21st Century: Using Genetic Information to Improve Health and Prevent Disease*, New York: Oxford University Press.

Davison, A., Barns, I. and Schibeci, R. (1997) 'Problematic publics: a critical review of surveys of public attitudes to biotechnology', *Science, Technology, and Human Values*, 22, 3: 317–48.

Dawkins, R. (1976) *The Selfish Gene*, Oxford: Oxford University Press.

Dayton, L. (1997a) 'Discovery of bowel cancer gene gives hope of prevention', *The Sydney Morning Herald*, 7 April: 6.

Dayton, L. (1997b) 'Long-dead soldier gives clue to deadliest epidemic', *The Sydney Morning Herald*, 22 March: 8.

Dayton, L. (1998) 'Researchers find gene that causes early-onset Parkinson's', *The Sydney Morning Herald*, 9 April: 5.

Debelle, P. (1998) 'Childless may demand cloning', *The Sydney Morning Herald*, 1 December: 5.

Diamond, J. (1997) *Guns, Germs and Steel: The Fates of Human Societies*, New York and London: W. W. Norton & Co.

Dickens, B. M., Pei, N. and Taylor, K. M. (1996) 'Legal and ethical issues in genetic testing and counselling for susceptibility to breast, ovarian and colon cancer', *Canadian Medical Association Journal*, 154, 6: 813–18.

Dienel, P. (1989) 'Contributing to social decision methodology: citizen reports on technological projects', in C. Vlek and G. Cuetkovich (eds), *Social Methodology for Technological Projects*, Dordrecht: Kluwer Academic Publishers.

Dikötter, F. (1998) *Imperfect Conceptions: Medical Knowledge, Birth Defects and Eugenics in China*, London: Hurst & Co.

Dobson, R. (1999) 'Science bites back', *The Australian*, 11 January: 16.

Dobson, A. and Lucardie, P. (1993) *The Politics of Nature: Explorations in Green Political Theory*, London: Routledge.

Dorman, J. S. and Mattison, D. R. (2000) 'Epidemiology, molecular biology, and public health', in M. J. Khoury, W. Burke, and E. J. Thomson (eds) *Genetics and Public Health in the 21st Century: Using Genetic Information to Improve Health and Prevent Disease*, New York: Oxford University Press.

Draper, E. (1991) *Risky Business: Genetic Testing and Exclusionary Practices in the Hazardous Workplace*, Cambridge: Cambridge University Press.

Draper, P. (1991) *Health through Public Policy: The Greening of Public Health*, London: Greenprint.

Dubos, R. (1959) *Mirage of Health: Utopias, Progress and Biological Change*, London: Allen & Unwin.

Dunkerley, D. and Glasner, P. (1998) 'Empowering the public? Citizens' juries and the new genetic technologies', *Critical Public Health*, 8, 3: 181–92.

Dunlop, R. E. and Catton, W. R. jr (1992/3) 'Towards an ecological sociology: the development, current status and probable future of environmental sociology', *The Annals of the International Institute of Sociology*, 3 (New Series): 263–84.

Durant, J., Hansen, A. and Bauer, M. (1996) 'Public understanding of the new genetics', in T. Marteau and M. Richards (eds) *The Troubled Helix: Social and Psychological Implications of the New Human Genetics*, Cambridge: Cambridge University Press.

Duster, T. (1990) *Backdoor to Eugenics*, London and New York: Routledge.

Eccleston, R. (1998) 'Revolution in the wings for pre-natal testing', *The Weekend Australian*, 28 February: 3.

Ellul, J. (1964) *The Technological Society*, New York: Vintage Books.

Elston, M. A. (1997) 'Introduction: The Sociology of Medical Science and Technology', in M. A. Elston (ed.) *The Sociology of Medical Science and Technology*, Oxford: Blackwell.

Ettorre, E. (1996) *The New Genetics Discourse in Finland: Exploring Experts' Views within Surveillance Medicine*, Helsinki: Suomen Kuntali-itto (Association of Finnish Metropolitan Authorities).

Ettorre, E. (2000) 'Reproductive genetics, gender and the body: "Please doctor, may I have a normal baby?"', *Sociology*, 34, 3: 403–20.

Evans, D. G. R., Blair, V., Greenhalgh, R., Hopwood, P. and Howell, A. (1994) 'The impact of genetic counselling on risk perception in women with a family history of breast cancer', *British Journal of Cancer*, 70: 934–8.

Ewing, T. (1997) 'Discovery of bowel cancer gene gives hope of prevention', *The Sydney Morning Herald*, 7 April: 6.

Ezrahi, Y. (1990) *The Descent of Icarus: Science and the Transformation of Contemporary Democracy*, Cambridge, MA: Harvard University Press.

Falk, P. (1994) *The Consuming Body*, London: Sage.

Fawcett, B. (2000) *Feminist Perspectives on Disability*, Harlow: Prentice Hall.

Featherstone, M. (1995) *Undoing Culture: Globalization, Postmodernism and Identity*, London: Sage.

Feldman, M. K. (1996) 'Genetic screening: not just another blood test', *Minnesota Medicine*, 79: 14–17.

Ferrari, J. (1997) 'Genetics hold key to beating cancer', *The Weekend Australian*, 8 March: 51.

Fineman, R. M. (1999) 'Qualifications of public health geneticists?', *Community Genetics*, 2: 113–14.

Finkler, K. (2000) *Experiencing the New Genetics: Family and Kinship on the Medical Frontier*, Philadelphia: University of Pennsylvania Press.

Foucault, M. (1976) *The Birth of the Clinic: An Archaeology of Medical Perception*, London: Tavistock.

Foucault, M. (1980) *The History of Sexuality, Volume 1: An Introduction*, New York: Vintage Books.

Foucault, M. (1986) *The Care of the Self*, New York: Pantheon.

Frenk, J. (1993) 'The new public health', *Annual Review of Public Health*, 14: 469–90.

Friedmann, T. (1994) *Gene Therapy: Fact and Fiction in Biology's New Approaches to Disease*, New York: Cold Spring Laboratory Press.

Fujimura, J. H. (1997) 'Constructing do-able problems in cancer research: articulating alignment', *Social Studies of Science*, 17: 257–93.

Galhardi, R. M. (1995) 'The impact of biotechnology on North–South trade', *Futures*, 27, 6: 641–56.

Garrett, L. (1994) *The Coming Plague: Newly Emerging Diseases in a World out of Balance*, New York: Farrar, Straus and Giroux.

Gaskell, G., Bauer, M. W., Durant, J. and Allum, N. C. (1999) 'Worlds apart? The reception of genetically modified foods in Europe and the US', *Science*, 284: 1442–4.

Geller, G. and Holtzman, N. A. (1995) 'A qualitative assessment of primary care physicians' perceptions about the ethical and social implications of offering genetic testing', *Qualitative Health Research*, 5, 1, 97–116.

Gene Watch (2000) www.genewatch.org/Press%20Releases/pr12.htm.

Genetic Services of Western Australia (1995) *Genetic Services of Western Australia*, Perth: GSWA.

Genetics Education Program (2000) *Genetics Resource Book: The Australian and New Zealand Directory of Genetics Support Groups, Services and Information*, Fifth Edition, 2000–2001, Sydney: Genetics Education Program of New South Wales.

Gert, B., Berger, E. M., Cahill, G. F., Clouser, K. D., Culver, C. M., Moeschler, J. B. and Singer, G. H. S. (1996) *Morality and the New Genetics: A Guide for Students and Health Care Providers*, Sudbury, MA: Jones and Barblett Publishers.

Gettig, E., Baker, T., Khoury, M. J., Bryan, J., Pierce, H., Puryear, M. and Thomson, E. (1999) 'Report on the Second National Conference on Genetics and Public Health, genetics and disease prevention: integrating genetics into public health policy, research and practice, Baltimore, Md., 6–8 December, 1999', *Community Genetics*, 2: 119–36.

Gibbs, D. (2000) 'Globalization, the bioscience industry and local environmental responses', *Global Environmental Change*, 10, 4: 245–57.

Giddens, A. (1991) *Modernity and Self-Identity: Self and Society in the Late Modern Age*, Cambridge: Polity.

Giddens, A. (1999) *The Reith Lectures*, http://news.bbc.uk

Gieryn, T. F. (1983) 'Boundary-work and the demarcation of science from non-science: strains and interests in professional ideologies of scientists', *American Sociological Review*, 48: 781–95.

Gieryn, T. F. (1995) 'Boundaries of science', in S. Jasanoff, G. E. Markle, J. C. Petersen and T. Pinch (eds) *Handbook of Science and Technology Studies*, Thousand Oaks: Sage.

Gill, M. and Richards, T. (1998) 'Meeting the challenge of genetic advance requires rigorous navigation between laboratory, clinic, and society', *British Medical Journal*, 316: 570.

Gillon, R. (1994) 'Ethics of genetic screening: the first report of the Nuffield Council on Bioethics', *Journal of Medical Ethics*, 20: 67–8.

Glasner, P. (2001) 'Rights or rituals: why juries can do more harm than good', in M. Pimbert and T. Wakeford (eds) *Deliberative Democracy and Citizen Empowerment*, Special Issue of 'PLA Notes', 40, February, International Institute for Environmental Development.

Glasner, P. and Dunkerley, P. (1999) 'The new genetics, public involvement, and citizens' juries: a Welsh case study', *Health, Risk and Society*, 1, 3: 313–24.

Goldberg, D. (1998) 'Cloning comes of age – just in time', *The Australian*, 27 July: 10.

Golden, F. (1999) 'Good eggs, bad eggs', Time.com, 153, 1 (January). (http://cgi.pathfinder.com/time/magazine/articles/0,3266,17683,00.html)

Goodell, R. (1986) 'How to kill a controversy: the case of recombinant DNA', in S. Friedman, M. Dunwoody and C. L. Rogers (eds) *Scientists and Journalists: Reporting Science as News*, New York: The Free Press.

Goodman, D. and Redclift, M. (1991) *Refashioning Nature: Food, Ecology and Culture*, London: Routledge, pp. 167–88.

Goonatilake, S. (1999) 'A post-European century in science', *Futures*, 31: 923–7.

Gostin, L. O. (1995) 'Genetic privacy', *Journal of Law, Medicine and Ethics*, 23: 320–30.

Goudsblom, J. (1986) 'Public health and the civilizing process', *The Milbank Quarterly*, 64, 2: 161–88.

Gould, S. J. (1998) 'Dolly's fashion and Louis's Passion', in M. C. Nussbaum and C. R. Sustein (eds) *Clones and Clones*, New York and London: W. W. Norton & Co.

Green, P. (1996) 'Gene therapy stalls fatal march of deadly asbestos disease', *The Australian*, 14 August: 7.

Griffiths, S. and Hunter, D. (eds) (1999) *Perspectives in Public Health*, Abingdon: Radcliffe Medical Press.

Guerinot, M. L. (2000) 'The green revolution strikes gold', *Science* (Washington), 287, 5451: 241–3.

Gupta, G. K. and Bianchi, D. W. (1997) 'Diagnosis for the practicing obstetrician', *Obstetric Gynecological Clinic North America*, 24, 1: 123–42.

Hajer, M. (1995) *The Politics of Environmental Discourse: Ecological Modernization and the Policy Processs*, Oxford: Clarendon Press.

Hamilton, M. P. (1972) *The New Genetics and the Future of Man*, Grand Rapids, MI: William B. Eerdmans Publishing Company.

Hannigan, J. A. (1995) *Environmental Sociology: A Social Constructionist Perspective*, London: Routedge.

Hansen, A. (1994) 'Journalistic practices and science reporting in the British press', *Public Understanding of Science*, 3, 2: 111–34.

Hansen, A. (2000) 'Claims-making and framing in British newspaper coverage of the "Brent Spar" controversy', in S. Allan, B. Adam and C. Carter (eds) *Environmental Risks and the Media*, London and New York: Routledge.

Hanson, M. J. (1999) 'Biotechnology and commodification within health care', *Journal of Medicine and Philosophy*, 24, 3: 267–87.

Harper, P. S. (1997) ' "Over the counter" genetic testing: lessons from cystic fibrosis carrier screening', in P. S. Harper and A. J. Clarke, *Genetics, Society and Clinical Practice*, Oxford: Bios Scientific Publishers.

Haraway, D. (1991) *Simians, Cyborgs and Women: The Reinvention of Nature*, London and New York: Routledge.

Harris, R. (1998) 'Genetic counselling and testing in Europe', *Journal of the Royal College of Physicians of London*, 32, 4: 335–8.

Harris, R., Harris, H. J., and Raeburn, J. A. (1999) 'Genetic services in Europe – primary care genetics is a priority for health care systems', in I. Nippert, H. Neitzel and G. Wolff (eds) *The New Genetics: From Research into Health Care, Social and Ethical Implications for Users and Providers*, Berlin and New York: Springer-Verlag.

Harris, T. (1997) 'Gene find brings hope for glaucoma sufferers', *The Weekend Australian*, 15–16 February: 52.

Harrison, B. (1971) *Drink and the Victorians: The Temperance Question in England, 1815–1872*, London: Faber.

Harvey, M. (1999) 'Cultivation and comprehension: how genetic modification irreversibility alters the human engagement with nature', *Sociological Research Online*, 4, 3.

Hatchwell, P. (1989) 'Opening Pandora's Box: the risks of genetically engineered organisms', *The Ecologist*, 14, 4: 130–6.

Hawkes, N. (1996) 'Gene find may lead to vaccine for malaria', *The Weekend Australian*, 12–13 October: 19.

Hawkes, N. and Rhodes, T. (1997) 'Human clones within 2 years', *The Weekend Australian*, 8 March: 15.

Hayes, R. (2000) 'In the pipeline: genetically modified humans?', *Multinational Monitor*, January: 29–34.

Hayflick, S. J. and Eiff, M. P. (1998) 'Role of primary care providers in the delivery of genetics services', *Community Genetics*, 1: 18–22.

Hecht, F. and Holmes, L. B. (1972) 'What we don't know about genetic counselling', *The New England Journal of Medicine*, 287, 9: 464–5.

Hedgecoe, A. M. (1999) 'Transforming genes: metaphors of information and language in modern genetics', *Science as Culture*, 8, 2: 209–29.

Heidegger, M. (1949) *Existence and Being*, Chicago: Regnery-Gateway.

Heidegger, M. (1977) *The Question Concerning Technology and Other Essays*, New York: Harper Torchbooks.

Henkel, J. (1995) 'Genetic engineering fast forwarding to future foods', *Consumer*, Washington: Federal Drugs Agency.

Hepburn, L. (1998) 'Genetic counselling: parental autonomy or acceptance of limits?', in M. Junker-Kenny and L. S. Cahill (eds) *The Ethics of Genetic Engineering*, London: SCM Press and Maryknoll, NY: Orbis Books.

Hereditary Disease Unit (1995) *Testing for Birth Defects in Pregnancy*, Perth: Health Department of Western Australia.

Hickman, B. (1998a) 'Cancer gene identified', *The Weekend Australian*, 28–9 March: 44.

Hickman, B. (1998b) 'New genes linked with cancer cells', *The Weekend Australian*, 20–1 June: 45.

Hickman, B. (1998c) 'Genetic link to disease', *The Weekend Australian*, 21–2 November: 39.

Hickman, B. (1999) 'Gene therapy for heart vessels' (Health), *The Weekend Australian*, 14–15 August: 7.

Hildt, E. and Graumann, S. (eds) (1999) *Genetics in Human Reproduction*, Aldershot: Ashgate.

Hileman, B. (1999) 'UK moratorium on biotech crops', *Chemical and Engineering News*, 24 May: 7.

Hilgartner, S. (1990) 'The dominant view of popularization: conceptual problems, political uses', *Social Studies of Science*, 20: 519–39.

Hill, A. and Michael, M. (1998) 'Engineering acceptance: representations of "the public" in debates on biotechnology', in P. Wheale, R. von Schomberg and P. Glasner (eds) *The Social Management of Genetic Engineering*, Aldershot: Ashgate.

Hill, K. and Dayton, L. (1998) 'How genetic secrets could cure the baby boomers', *The Sydney Morning Herald*, 31 March: 1, 4.

Hill, S. (1988) *The Tragedy of Technology: Human Liberation Versus Domination in the Late Twentieth Century*, London: Pluto.

Hill, S. (1994) *Managing Sickle Cell Disease in Low-Income Families*, Philadelphia: Temple University Press.

Ho, M. W., Traavik, T., Olsvik, O., Tappeser, B., Howard, C. V. , von Weizsacker, C. and McGavin, G. C. (1998) 'Gene technology and gene ecology of infectious diseases', *Microbial Ecology in Health and Disease*, 10: 33–59.

Hoban, T. J. (1999) 'Consumer acceptance of biotechnology in the United States and Japan', *Food Technology*, 53, 5: 50–3.

Holiday, R. (1990) *Philosophical Transactions of the Royal Society of London*, B326.

Holdredge, C. (1996) *A Question of Genes: Understanding Life in Context*, Hudson, New York: Lindisfarne Press.

Holland, W.W., Detels, R. Knox, G.E. and Breeze, E. (1984) *Oxford Textbook of Public Health*, Oxford: Oxford University Press.

Holtzman, N. A. and Marteau, T. M. (2000) 'Will genetics revolutionize medicine?', *The New England Journal of Medicine*, 343, 2: 141–4.

Horgan, J. (1993) 'Eugenics revisited', *Scientific American*, June: 92–100.

Hoy, A. (1997) 'Experts rush to embrace cloning process', *The Sydney Morning Herald*, 25 February: 8.

Hsia, Y. E. (1974) 'Choosing my children's genes: genetic counseling', in M. Lipkin and P. T. Rowley (eds), *Genetic Responsibility: On Choosing Our Children's Genes*, New York and London: Plenum Press.

Hubbard, R. and Wald, E. (1997) *Exploding the Gene Myth: How Genetic Information is Produced and Manipulated By Scientists, Physicians, Employers, Insurance Companies, Educators and Law Enforcers*, Boston: Beacon Press.

Hughes, T. P. (1983) *Networks of Power: Electric Supply Systems in the US, England and Germany, 1880–1930*, Baltimore: Johns Hopkins University Press.

Huibers, A. K. and van 't Spijker, A. (1998) 'The autonomy paradox: predictive genetic testing and autonomy: three essential problems', *Patient Education and Counselling*, 35, 1: 53–62.

Human Genetics Commission (undated) *Whose Hands on Your Genes? A Discussion Document on the Storage, Protection and Use of Personal Genetic Information*, London: HGC (www.hgc.gov.uk).

Hume, J. (1996) 'Disability, feminism and eugenics', *Quad Wrangle*, Autumn: 4–6.

Institute of Medicine (1997) *America's Vital Interest in Global Health*, Washington, DC: National Academy Press.

Irwin, A., Rothstein, H., Yearley, S. and McCarthy, E. (1997) 'Regulatory science – towards a sociological framework', *Futures*, 29, 1: 17–31.

Isaacson, W. (1999) 'The biotech century', Time.com, 153, 1 (January 11): 1–2.

Jackson, J. F. (1996) *Genetics and You*, Totowa, NJ: Humana Press.

Jaroff, L. (1991) *The New Genetics*, Knoxville, TN: The Grand Rounds Press (Whittle Direct Books).

Jessop, B. (1999) 'Reflections on globalization and its (il)logic(s)', P. Dicken *et al.* (eds) *The Logic of Globalization*, London and New York: Routledge.

Joffe, H. (1999) *Risk and 'the Other'*, Cambridge: Cambridge University Press.

Johnson, R. (undated) 'Western Australian Government's response to WACAMAC's recommendations', in Citizenship and Multicultural

Interests, *The Way Forward, Citizenship: Building a Shared Future*. A Response to the Citizenship Discussion Paper, Perth: The Government of Western Australia.

Joss, S. (1995) 'Evaluating consensus conferences: necessity or luxury?', in S. Joss and J. Durant (eds) *Public Participation in Science: The Role of Consensus Conferences in Europe*, London: Science Museum.

Joss, S. and Durant, J. (eds) (1995) *Public Participation in Science: The Role of Consensus Conferences in Europe*, London: Science Museum.

Kallianes, V. and Rubenfeld, P. (1997) 'Disabled women and reproductive rights', *Disability and Society*, 12, 2: 203–21.

Kaplan, J. M. (2000) *The Limits and Lies of Human Genetic Research: Dangers for Social Policy*, London and New York: Routledge.

Karpf, A. (1988) *Doctoring the Media: The Reporting of Health and Medicine*, London and New York: Routledge.

Katz Rothman, B. (1998) *Genetic Maps and Human Imaginations: The Limits of Science in Understanding Who We Are*, New York and London: W. W. Norton & Co.

Kearney, M. (1995) 'The local and the global: the anthropology of globalization and transnationalism', *Annual Review of Anthropology*, 24: 547–65.

Keller, E. F. (1992) 'Nature, nurture, and the Human Genome Project', in D. J. Kevles and L. Hood (eds) *The Code of Codes: Scientific and Social Issues in the Human Genome Project*, Cambridge, MA and London: Harvard University Press.

Keller, E. F. (2000) *The Century of the Gene*, Cambridge, MA and London: Harvard University Press.

Kenen, R. H. (1986) 'Growing pains of a new health care field: genetic counselling in Australia and the United States', *Australian Journal of Social Issues*, 21, 3: 172–82.

Kenen, R. H. (1997) 'Opportunities and impediments for a consolidating and expanding profession: genetic counseling in the United States', *Social Science and Medicine*, 45, 9: 1377–86.

Kenen, R. H. and Smith, A. C. M. (1995) 'Genetic counseling for the next 25 years: models for the future', *Journal of Genetic Counseling*, 4, 2: 115–24.

Kerin, J. (2001) 'See your own death through DNA', *The Australian*, 7 June: 3.

Kerr, A. and Cunningham-Burley, S. (2000) 'On ambivalence and risk: reflexive modernity and the new human genetics', *Sociology*, 34, 2: 283–304.

Kerr, A., Cunningham-Burley, S. and Amos, A. (1997) 'The new genetics: professionals' discursive boundaries', *Sociological Review*, 45: 279–303.

Kerr, A., Cunningham-Burley, S. and Amos, A. (1998a) 'The new genetics and health: mobilizing lay expertise', *Public Understanding of Science*, 7, 1: 41–60.

Kerr, A., Cunningham-Burley, S. and Amos, A. (1998b) 'Drawing the line: an analysis of lay people's discussions about the new genetics', *Public Understanding of Science*, 7, 2: 113–33.

Kerr, A., Cunningham-Burley, S. and Amos, A. (1998c) 'Eugenics and the new genetics in Britain: examining contemporary professionals' accounts', *Science, Technology and Human Values*, 23, 2: 175–99.

Kevles, D. J. (1995) *In the Name of Eugenics: Genetics and the Uses of Human Heredity*, Cambridge, MA and London: Harvard University Press.

Khoury, M. J. (1996) 'From genes to public health: the applications of genetic technology in disease prevention', *American Journal of Public Health*, 86, 12: 1717–22.

Khoury, M. J. (1998) 'The Human Genome Epidemiology Network (HuGE Net)' [conference abstract], in M. J. Khoury, M. Puryear, E. Thomson and J. Bryan, 'Translating advances in human genetics into disease prevention and health promotion', *Community Genetics*, 1: 93–108.

Khoury, M. J., Burke, W. and Thomson, E. J. (eds) (2000) *Genetics and Public Health in the 21st Century: Using Genetic Information to Improve Health and Prevent Disease*, New York: Oxford University Press.

Khoury, M. J., Puryear, M., Thomson, E. and Bryan, J. (1998) 'Translating advances in human genetics into disease prevention and health promotion', *Community Genetics*, 1: 93–108.

Kidd, J. S. and Kidd, R. A. (1999) *Life Lines: The Story of the New Genetics*, New York: Facts On File, Inc.

King, D. (1995) 'The state of eugenics', *New Statesman and Society*, 25 August: 25–6.

Kinmonth, A. L., Reinhard, J., Bobrow, M. and Pauker, S. (1998) 'The new genetics: implications for clinical services in Britain and the United States', *British Medical Journal*, 316, 7133: 767–70.

Kitto, H. D. F. (1957) *The Greeks*, London: Pelican.

Koch, L. (1999) 'Predictive genetic medicine – a new concept of disease', in E. Hildt and S. Graumann (eds) *Genetics in Human Reproduction*, Aldershot: Ashgate.

Kolata, G. (1997) *Clone: The Road to Dolly and the Path Ahead*, London: Allen Lane.

Koshland, D. (2000) 'Ethics and safety', in G. Stock and J. Campbell *Engineering the Human Germline: An Exploration of the Science and Ethics of Altering the Genes We Pass to Our Children*, New York and Oxford: Oxford University Press.

Krieger, N. (1999) 'Sticky webs, hungry spiders, buzzing flies, and fractal metaphors: on the misleading juxtaposition of "risk factor" versus "social" epidemiology,' *Journal of Epidemiological Community Health*, 53: 678–80.

Krieger, N. (2000) 'Epidemiology and social sciences: towards a critical reengagement in the 21st century', *Epidemiologic Reviews*, 22, 1: 155–63.

Larriera, A. (1996) 'Discovery of mutant gene offers HIV hope', *The Sydney Morning Herald*, 28 September: 6.

Lasch, C. (1991) *True and Only Heaven: Progress and its Critics*, New York and London: W. W. Norton & Co.

Lash, S. and Urry, J. (1994) *Economies of Signs and Space*, London: Sage.

Latour, B. (1986) 'Visualization and cognition: thinking with eyes and hands', in H. Kuklick and E. Long (eds) *Knowledge and Society: Studies in the Sociology of Culture Past and Present*, A Research Annual, Greenwich, CT and London: JAI Press Inc.

Latour, B. (1987) *Science in Action*, Milton-Keynes: Open University Press.

Latour, B. (1992) 'Where are the missing masses?', in W. Bijker and J. Law (eds) *Shaping Technology/Building Society*, Cambridge, MA: MIT Press.

Latour, B. (1993) *We Have Never Been Modern*, Hemel Hempstead: Harvester Wheatsheaf.

Latour, B. (1997) *The Pasteurization of French Society, with Irreductions*, Cambridge, MA: Harvard University Press.

Latour, B. and Woolar, S. (1986) *Laboratory Life*, 2nd edition, Princeton, NJ: Princeton University Press.

Law, J. (2000) *Networks, Relations, Cyborgs: On the Social Study of Technology*, Online paper published by the Centre for Science Studies, Lancaster University, UK.

Le Vay, S. (1996) *Queer Science: The Use and Abuse of Research into Homosexuality*, Cambridge, MA: MIT Press.

Leech, G. (1998a) 'Vaccine warrior', *The Australian*, 18 May: 10.

Leech, G. (1998b) 'Resistance to drugs cracks', *The Weekend Australian*, 18–19 July: 40.

Leigh-Starr, S. (1991) 'Power, technology and the phenomenology of conventions: on being allergic to onions', in J. Law (ed.) *A Sociology of Monsters: Essays on Power, Technology and Domination*, Sociological Review Monograph 38, London: Macmillan.

Leonard, C. O., Chase, G. A. and Childs, B. (1972) 'Genetic counseling: a consumer's view', *The New England Journal of Medicine*, 287, 9: 433–9.

Leopold, A. (1966) *A Sand County Almanac*, New York: Ballantine Books.

Levine, H. G. (1978) 'The discovery of addiction: changing conceptions of habitual drunkenness in America', *Journal of Studies on Alcohol*, 39: 143–74.

Lewenstein, B. V. (1995) 'Science and media', in S. Jasanoff, G. E. Markle, J. C. Petersen and T. Pinch (eds) *Handbook of Science and Technology Studies*, Thousand Oaks: Sage.

Limoges, C. (1994) '*Errare Humanum Est* Do genetic errors have a future?', in C. F. Cranor (ed.) *Are Genes Us? The Social Consequences of the New Genetics*, New Brunswick, NJ: Rutgers University Press.

Lippman, A. (1992) 'Mother matters: a fresh look at prenatal genetic testing', *Issues in Reproductive and Genetic Engineering*, 5, 2: 141–54.

Lippman, A. (1999) 'Embodied knowledge and making sense of prenatal diagnosis', *Journal of Genetic Counseling*, 8, 5: 255–73.

Little, W., Fowler, H.W., Coulson, J.S., Onions, C.T. and Friedrichsen, G.W.S. (1973) *The Shorter Oxford English Dictionary on Historic Principles*, Oxford: Clarendon Press.

Lloyd, E. A. (1994) 'Normality and variation: the Human Genome Project and the ideal human type', in C. F. Cranor (ed.) *Are Genes Us? The Social Consequences of the New Genetics*, New Brunswick, NJ: Rutgers University Press.

Logan, R. A. (1991) 'Popularization versus secularization: media coverage of health', in L. Wilkins and P. Patterson (eds) *Risky Business: Communicating Issues of Science, Risk and Public Policy*, New York: Greenwood.

Love, R. (1996) 'Knowing your genes', *Public Understanding of Science*, 5, 1: 21–7.

Lunn, S. (1998) 'Cloners consider our wants and needs', *The Australian*, 15 April: 5.

Lupton, D. (1995) *The Imperative of Health: Public Health and the Regulated Body*, London: Sage.

Lupton, D. (2000) 'The social construction of the body', in G. Albrecht, R. Fitzpatrick and S. C. Scrimshaw (eds) *Handbook of Social Studies in Health and Medicine*, London: Sage.

McCarthy, A. (2000) 'Pharmacogenetics: implications for drug development, patients and society', *New Genetics and Society*, 19, 2: 135–43.

Macdonald, K. G., Doan, B., Kelner, M. and Taylor, K. M. (1996) 'A sociobehavioural perspective on genetic testing and counselling for heritable breast, ovarian and colon cancer', *Candian Medical Association Journal*, 145, 4: 457–64.

McGuirk, R. (1997) 'Potential exists for early Alzheimer's cure', *The Weekend Australian*, 13 September: 50.

McKeown, T. J. (1976) *The Role of Medicine: Dream, Mirage or Nemesis*, London: Nuffield Provincial Hospitals Trust.

McNally, R. and Wheale, P. (1998) 'The consequences of modern genetic engineering: patents, "nomads" and the "bio-industrial complex"', in P.

Wheale, R. von Schomberg and P. Glasner (eds) *The Social Management of Genetic Engineering*, Aldershot: Ashgate.

Mackta, J. and Weiss, J. O. (1994) 'The role of genetic support groups', *Journal of Obstetric, Gynecologic and Neonatal Nursing*, 23, 6: 519–23.

Mahowald, M. B. (1994) 'Reproductive genetics and gender justice', in K. H. Rothenberg and E. J. Thomson (eds) *Women and Prenatal Testing: Facing the Challenges of Genetic Technology*, Columbus: Ohio State University Press.

Mahowald, M. B. (1996) 'A feminist standpoint for genetics', *The Journal of Clinical Ethics*, 7, 4: 333–40.

Mahowald, M. B. (1997) 'Gender justice in genetics', *Women's Health Issues*, 7, 4: 230–3.

Mahowald, M. B. (2000) *Genes, Women, Equality*, New York: Oxford University Press.

Mahowald, M. B., Levinson, D. and Cassel, C., Lemke, A., Ober, C., Bowman, J., Le Beau, M., Ravin A. and Times, M. (1996) 'The new genetics and women', *The Milbank Quarterly*, 74, 2: 239–83.

Malinowski, M. J. (1994) 'Coming into being: law, ethics, and the practice of prenatal genetic screening', *The Hastings Law Journal*, 45, 6: 1435–526.

Markel, H. (1992) 'The stigma of disease: implications of genetic screening', *American Journal of Medicine*, 93: 209–15.

Marteau, T. M. and Croyle, R. T. (1998) 'Psychological responses to genetic testing', *British Medical Journal*, 316 : 693–6.

Marteau, T., Drake, H. and Bobrow, M. (1994) 'Counselling following diagnosis of a fetal abnormality: the differing approaches of obstetricians, clinical geneticists, and genetic nurses', *Journal of Medical Genetics*, 31: 864–7.

Martin, E. (1994) *Flexible Bodies: Tracking Immunity in American Culture from the Days of Polio to the Age of AIDS*, Boston, MA: Beacon Press.

Martin, L. H., Gutman, H. and Hutton, P. H. (1988) *Technologies of the Self: A Seminar with Michel Foucault*, London: Tavistock.

Martin, P. (1995) 'The American gene therapy industry and the social shaping of a new technology', *The Genetic Engineer and Biotechnologist*, 15: 155–67.

Martin, P. (1998) 'From eugenics to therapeutics: the impact of opposition on the development of gene therapy in the USA', in P. Wheale, R. von Schomberg and P. Glasner (eds) *The Social Management of Genetic Engineering*, Aldershot: Ashgate.

Martin, P. (1999) 'Genes as drugs: the social shaping of gene therapy and the reconstruction of genetic disease,' *Sociology of Health and Illness*, 21, 5: 517–38.

Martin, P. and Kaye, J. (2000) 'The use of large biological sample collections in genetics research: issues for public policy', *New Genetics and Society*, 19, 2: 165–91.

Marx, K. (1967) *Capital: A Critique of Political Economy*, New York: International.

Mayer, I. and Geurts, J. (1998) 'Consensus conferences as participatory policy analysis: a methodological contribution to the social management of technology', in P. Wheale, R. von Schomberg and P. Glasner (eds) *The Social Management of Genetic Engineering*, Aldershot: Ashgate.

Mead, A. (1995) 'Letter to Darryl Macer', posted on Native-L, www.nativenet.uthscsa.edu/archive/al/

Mead, A. (1996) 'Genealogy, sacredness and the commodities market', *Cultural Survival Quarterly*, 20: 46–51.

Meek, J. (2000) 'Scientists hail gene therapy that fights cancer tumours', *Guardian Weekly*, 3–9 August: 9.

Mellor, P. and Shilling, C. (1997) *Re-forming the Body: Religion, Community and Modernity*, London: Sage.

Melucci, A. (1989) *Nomads of the Present: Social Movements and Individual Needs in Contemporary Society*, London: Hutchinson Radius.

Mendelson, J. (1998) 'Roudup; the world's biggest-selling herbicide', *The Ecologist*, 28, 5: 270–5.

Meredith, H. (2000) 'Biotechnology is the next great wave', *The Australian Financial Review*, 13 July : 3.

Michie, S. and Marteau, T. (1999) 'Genetic counselling: some issues of theory and practice', in T. Marteau and M. Richards (eds) *The Troubled Helix: Social and Psychological Implications of the New Human Genetics*, Cambridge: Cambridge University Press.

Milio, N. (1986) *Promoting Health through Public Policy*, Ottawa: Canadian Public Health Association.

Miller, M. M. and Riechert, B. P. (2000) 'Interest group strategies and journalistic norms: news media framing of environmental issues', in S. Allan, B. Adam and C. Carter (eds) *Environmental Risks and the Media*, London and New York: Routledge.

Miringoff, M.-L. (1991) *The Social Costs of Genetic Welfare*, New Brunswick, NJ: Rutgers University Press.

Mitchell, S. (2000) 'Moves on e-health records put privacy issues in focus', *The Australian*, 18 July: 35.

Mittman, H. S., Penchaszadeh, V. B. and Secundy, M. G. (1998) 'The national dialogue on genetics, College Park, Maryland, March 21–22, 1998', *Community Genetics*, 1, 3: 115–200.

Mosley, W. H., Bobadilla, J. L. and Jamison, D. T. (1993) 'The health transition: implications for health policy in developing countries', in D. T. Jamison, W. H. Mosley, A. R. Measham and J. L. Bobadilla (eds)

Disease Control Priorities in Developing Countries, New York: Oxford Medical Publications.

Mumford, L. (1934) *Technics and Civilization*, New York: Harcourt Brace.

Murcott, A. (1999) ' "Not science but PR": GM food and the making of a considered sociology', *Sociology Research Online*, 4, 3.

Murray, C. J. L. and Lopez, A. D. (1996) 'Evidence-based health policy: lessons from the global burden of disease study', *Science*, 274: 740–3.

Nash, J. M. (1997) 'The age of cloning: a line has been crossed, and reproductive biology will never be the same for people or for sheep', *Time*, 10 March, 149, 10: 62–5.

Nason, D. (1994) 'Tickner warns over Aboriginal gene sampling', *The Australian*, 25 January: 3.

Navaro, V. (1993) *Dangerous to Your Own Health: Capitalism in Health Care*, New York: Monthly Review Press.

Navaro, V. (1998) 'Comment: whose globalization?', *American Journal of Public Health*, 88: 742.

Nazroo, J. Y. (1998) 'Genetic, cultural or socio-economic vulnerability? Explaining ethnic inequalities in health', *Sociology of Health and Illness*, 20: 714–34.

Nelkin, D. (1985) 'Managing biomedical news', *Social Research*, 52, 3: 625–46.

Nelkin, D. (1987) *Selling Science: How the Press Covers Science and Technology*, New York: W. H. Freeman & Co.

Nelkin, D. (1994) 'Promotional metaphors and their popular appeal', *Public Understanding of Science*, 3, 1: 25–31.

Nelkin, D. (1995) 'Forms of intrusion: comparing resistance to information technology and biotechnology in the USA', in M. Bauer (ed.) *Resistance to New Technology: Nuclear Power, Information Technology and Biotechnology*, Cambridge: Cambridge University Press.

Nelkin, D. and Andrews, L. (1999) 'DNA identification and surveillance creep', in P. Conrad and J. Gabe (eds) *Sociological Perspectives on the New Genetics*, Oxford: Blackwell.

Nelkin, D. and Lindee, M. S. (1995) *The DNA Mystique: The Gene as a Cultural Icon*, New York: W. H. Freeman.

Newell, C. (1999a) 'The social nature of disability, disease and genetics: a response to Gillam, Persson, Holtug, Draper and Chadwick', *Journal of Medical Ethics*, 25: 172–5.

Newell, C. (1999b) ' "Disabling health systems" ', *interaction*, 12, 4: 13–16.

Newell, C. (1999c) 'Critical reflections on disability, difference and the new genetics', in G. O'Sullivan, E. Sharman and S. Short (eds) *Goodbye Normal Gene: Confronting the Genetic Revolution*, Annandale: Pluto Press Australia Ltd. and Public Health Association of Australia Inc.

NIAID Fact Sheet (1998) 'Summary of the blue ribbon panel on malaria vaccine development', www.niaid.nih.gov/dmid/panel.htm

Nielsen, L. (1999) 'The Icelandic health sector data base: legal and ethical considerations', in T. A. Caulfield and B. Williams-Jones (eds) *The Commercialization of Genetic Research: Ethical, Legal, and Policy Issues*, Dordrecht: Kluwer/Plenum Publishers.

Nippert, I., Neitzel, H. and Wolff, G. (eds) (1999) *The New Genetics: From Research into Health Care, Social and Ethical Implications for Users and Providers*, Berlin and Heidelberg, NY: Springer.

Nossal, G. (1998) 'The dawning of a new age of therapy', *The Sydney Morning Herald*, 31 March: 4.

Nottingham, S. (1998) *Eat Your Genes: How Genetically Modified Food is Entering Our Diet*, London and New York: Zed Books.

Novas, C. and Rose, N. (2000) 'Genetic risk and the birth of the somatic individual', *Economy and Society*, 29, 4: 485–513.

O'Sullivan, G., Sharman, E. and Short, S. (1999) *Goodbye Normal Gene: Confronting the Genetic Revolution*, Annandale: Pluto Press and Public Health Association of Australia Inc.

Oudshoorn, N. (1994) *Beyond the Natural Body: An Archaelogy of Sex Hormones*, London and New York: Routledge.

Parens, E. (1998) 'Is better always good? The Enhancement Project', in E. Parens (ed.) *Enhancing Human Traits: Ethical and Social Implications*, Washington, DC: Georgetown University Press.

Parens, E. and Asch, A. (1999) 'The disability rights critique of prenatal genetic testing', *The Hastings Center Report*, 29, 5: 1–35.

Parisi, L. and Terranova, T. (2000) 'Heat-Death [Part 1]: emergence and control in genetic engineering and artificial life', *Ctheory Theory, Technology and Culture*, 23, 1–2, Article 84[I] 05/10/00.

Paul, D. (1994) 'Eugenic anxieties, social realities, and political choices', in C. F. Cranor (ed.) *Are Genes Us? The Social Consequences of the New Genetics*, New Brunswick, NJ: Rutgers University Press.

Peters, J. A., Djurdjinovic, L. and Baker, D. (1999) 'The genetic self: the Human Genome Project, Genetic Counseling, and family therapy', *Families, Systems and Health*, 17, 1: 5–25.

Petersen, A. (1994) *In a Critical Condition: Health and Power Relations in Australia*, Sydney: Allen & Unwin.

Petersen, A. (1998a) 'The new genetics and the politics of public health', *Critical Public Health*, 8, 1: 59–71.

Petersen, A. (1998b) *Unmasking the Masculine: 'Men' and 'Identity' in a Sceptical Age*, London: Sage.

Petersen, A. (1999) 'The portrayal of research into genetic-based differences of sex and sexual orientation: a study of "popular" science journals, 1980 to 1997', *Journal of Communication Inquiry*, 23, 2: 163–82.

Petersen, A. (2001) 'Biofantasies: genetics and medicine in the print news media', *Social Science and Medicine*, 52, 8: 1255–68.

Petersen, A. and Bunton, R. (eds) (1997) *Foucault, Health and Medicine*, London and New York: Routledge.

Petersen, A. and Lupton, D. (1996) *The New Public Health: Health and Self in the Age of Risk*, London: Sage and Sydney: Allen & Unwin.

Petersen, A., Barns, I., Dudley, J. and Harris, P. (1999) *Poststructuralism, Citizenship and Social Policy*, London and New York: Routledge.

Pinch, T. J. and Bijker, W. E. (1984) 'The social construction of facts and artifacts – how the sociology of science and sociology of technology might benefit each other', *Social Studies of Science*, 14, 3: 399–441.

Pippin, R. B. (1994) 'On the notion of technology as ideology: prospects', in Y. Ezrahi, E. Mendelsohn and H. Segal (eds) *Technology, Pessimism and Postmodernism*, Dordrecht: Kluwer Academic Publishers.

Plant, R. (1974) *Community and Ideology: An Essay in Applied Social Philosophy*, London: Routledge and Kegan Paul.

Poortman, Y. (1999) 'The European Alliance of Genetic Support Groups, their ethical code and the provision of genetic services', in I. Nippert, H. Neitzel and G. Wolff (eds) *The New Genetics: From Research into Health Care, Social and Ethical Implications for Users and Providers*, Berlin and New York: Springer-Verlag.

Porter, D. (1997) 'Public health', in W. F. Bynum and R. Porter (eds) *Companion Encyclopedia of the History of Medicine*, vol. 2, London and New York: Routledge.

Porter, D. and Porter, R. (1988) 'The enforcement of health', in E. Fee and D. Fox (eds) *AIDS: The Burden of History*, Berkeley, CA: University of California Press.

Priest, S. H. (1994) 'Structuring public debate on biotechnology', *Science Communication*, 16, 2: 166–79.

Prout, A. (1996) 'Actor-network theory, technology and medical sociology: an illustrative example of the metered dose inhaler', *Sociology of Health and Illness*, 18, 2: 198–219.

Pullen, I. M. (1990) 'Patients, families and genetic information', in E. Sutherland and A. McCall Smith (eds) *Family Rights: Family Law and Medical Advance*, Edinburgh: Edinburgh University Press.

Rabinow, P. (1989) *French Modern: Norms and Forms of the Social Environment*, Cambridge, MA: MIT Press.

Rabinow, P. (1992) 'Artificiality and enlightenment: from sociobiology to biosociality', in J. Crary and S. Kwinter (eds) *Incorporations*, New York: Urzone.

Radford, T. (2001) 'Human genome code deepens mystery of life', *The Guardian Weekly*, 164, 8: 1.

Rajchman, J. (1984) 'The story of Foucault's history', *Social Text*, 8: 15.

Randall, V.R. (2000) 'Who owns the human genetic code?: annotated bibliography', www.udayton.edu~health/05bioethics/00ammons.htm

Rapp, R. (1988) 'Chromosomes and communication: the discourse of genetic counselling', *Medical Anthropology Quarterly*, 2, 2: 143–57.

Rapp, R. (1999) *Testing Women, Testing the Fetus: The Social Impact of Amniocentesis in America*, New York and London: Routledge.

Reiner, V. (1999) 'Ataxia challenge co-ordinated', *The Weekend Australian*, 17 April: 39.

Reiss, M. J. and Straughan, R. (1996) *Improving Nature? The Science and Ethics of Genetic Engineering*, Cambridge: Cambridge University Press.

Renn, O., Webler, T. and Wiedmann, P. (1995) 'A need for discourse on citizen participation: objectives and structure of the book' in O. Renn, T. Webler and P. Wiedmann (eds) *Fairness and Competence in Citizen Participation: Evaluating Models of Environmental Discourse*, Dordrecht: Kluwer Academic Publishers.

Resta, R. G. (1997) 'Eugenics and nondirectiveness in genetic counselling', *Journal of Genetic Counseling*, 6, 2: 255–8.

Rheinberger, H.-J. (1995) 'Beyond nature and culture: a note on medicine in the age of molecular biology', *Science in Context*, 8, 1: 249–63.

Ridley, M. (1999) *Genome: The Autobiography of a Species in 23 Chapters*, London: Fourth Estate.

Rifkin, J. (1998) *The Biotech Century: How Genetic Commerce Will Change the World*, London: Phoenix.

Ritzer, G. (1993) *The McDonaldization of Society*, London: Sage.

Roberts, J. (1993) 'Global project under way to sample genetic diversity', *Nature*, 361: 675.

Robertson, R. (1992) *Globalization*, London: Sage.

Robin, R. (2001) 'Endgame in a germ war', *Candian Business*, 19 February: 43–4.

Robotham, J. (1999) 'Grow a new limb using your own cells', *The Sydney Morning Herald*, 3 April: 1.

Rock, P. J. (1996) 'Eugenics and euthanasia: a cause for concern for disabled people, particularly disabled women', *Disability and Society*, 11, 1: 121–7.

Rona, R. J., Beech, R., Mandalla, S., Donnai, D., Kingston, H., Harris, R., Wilson, O., Axtell, C., Swan, A. V. and Kavanagh, F. (1994) 'The influence of genetic counselling in the era of DNA testing on knowledge, reproductive intentions and psychological wellbeing', *Clinical Genetics*, 46: 198–204.

Rose, H. (2001) *The Commodification of Bioinformation: The Icelandic Health Sector Database*, London: The Wellcome Trust.

Rose, N. (1989) *Governing the Soul: The Shaping of the Private Self*, London and New York: Routledge.

Rose, N. (1999) *Powers of Freedom: Reframing Political Thought*, Cambridge: Cambridge University Press.

Rose, N. and Miller, P. (1992) 'Political power beyond the state: problematics of government', *British Journal of Sociology*, 43, 2: 173–205.

Rose, P. (1999) 'Counselling techniques', in P. W. Rose and A. Lucassen, *Practical Genetics for Primary Care*, Oxford and New York: Oxford University Press.

Rose, P. W. and Lucassen, A. (1999) *Practical Genetics for Primary Care*, Oxford and New York: Oxford University Press.

Rosen, G. (1958) *A History of Public Health*, New York: MD Publications.

Rothenberg, K. H. and Thomson, E. J. (1994) *Women and Prenatal Testing: Facing the Challenges of Genetic Technology*, Columbus: Ohio State University Press.

Russell, D. A. (1999) 'Feasibility of antibody production in plants for human therapeutic use', *Current Topics in Microbiology and Immunology*, 240: 119–38.

Russo, E. and Cove, D. (1995) *Genetic Engineering: Dreams and Nightmares*, Oxford: W. H. Freeman.

Samet, J. M. and Bailey, L. A. (1997) 'Environmental population screening', in M. A. Rothstein (ed.) *Genetic Secrets: Protecting Privacy and Confidentiality in the Genetic Era*, New Haven and London: Yale University Press.

Sarkar, S. (1998) *Genetics and Reductionism*, Cambridge: Cambridge University Press.

Sawicki, J. (1991) *Disciplining Foucault: Feminism, Power, and the Body*, London and New York: Routledge.

Scrinis, G. (1995) *Colonizing the Seed: Genetic Engineering and Techno-industrial Agriculture*, Melbourne: Friends of the Earth.

Segal, H. P. (1994) 'Technology, pessimism, and postmodernism: introduction', in Y. Ezrahi, E. Mendelsohn and H. Segal (eds) *Technology, Pessimism and Postmodernism*, Dordrecht: Kluwer Academic Publishers.

Shakespeare, T. (1995) 'Back to the future? New genetics and disabled people', *Critical Social Policy*, 15, 2/3: 22–35.

Shakespeare, T. (1998) 'Choices and rights: eugenics, genetics and disability equality', *Disability and Society*, 13, 5: 665–81.

Shakespeare, T. (1999a) 'Losing the plot? Medical and activist discourses of the contemporary genetics and disability', in P. Conrad and J. Gabe (eds), *Sociological Perspectives on the New Genetics*, Oxford: Blackwell.

Shakespeare, T. (1999b) 'Manifesto for genetic justice', *Social Alternatives*, 18, 1: 29–32.

Shakespeare, T. and Erickson, M. (2000) 'Different strokes: beyond biological determinism and social constructionism', in H. Rose and S. Rose (eds) *Alas, Poor Darwin: Arguments Against Evolutionary Psychology*, London: Jonathan Cape.

Shildrick, M. (1997) *Leaky Bodies: Feminism, Postmodernism and (Bio)Ethics*, London and New York: Routledge.

Shiva, V. (1992) The seed and the earth: women, ecology and biotechnology', *The Ecologist*, 22, 1.

Shiva, V. (1993) *Monocultures of the Mind: Biodiversity, Biotechnology and the Third World*, Penang: Third World Network.

Shiva, V. and Dankelman, I. (1992) 'Women and biological diversity: lessons from the Indian Himalaya', in D. Cooper R. Vellve and H. Hobbelink (eds) *Growing Diversity: Genetic Resources and local Food Security*, London: ITDG Publishing.

Shulman, S. (1999) *Owning the Future*, Boston: Houghton Mifflin.

Silver, L. M. (1998) *Remaking Eden: Cloning and Beyond in a Brave New World*, London: Weidenfeld & Nicolson.

Silver, L. M. (2000) 'Reprogenetics: how reproductive and genetic technologies will be combined to provide new opportunities for people to reach their reproductive goals', in G. Stock and J. Campbell (eds) *Engineering the Human Germline: An Exploration of the Science and Ethics of Altering the Genes We Pass to Our Children*, New York and Oxford: Oxford University Press.

Simopolous, A. P., Herbert, V. and Jacobson, B. (1993) *Genetic Nutrition: Designing a Diet Based on Your Family Medical History*, New York: Macmillan.

Smith, D. (1997) 'Send in the clones', *The Sydney Morning Herald*, 1 March: 36.

Smith, D. (1998a) 'Made to order', *The Sydney Morning Herald*, 18 December: 11.

Smith, D. (1998b) 'Maverick will clone his wife', *The Sydney Morning Herald*, 18 December: 11.

Sneddon, R. (2000) 'The challenge of pharmacogenetics and pharmacogenomics', *New Genetics and Society*, 19, 2: 145–64.

Sobchack, V. (1995) 'Beating the meat/surviving the text, or how to get out of this century alive', *Body and Society*, 1, 3–4: 205–14.

Spaagaren, G. and Mol, A. P. J. (1992) 'Sociology, environment and modernity: ecological modernization as a theory of social change', *Society and Natural Resources*, 5: 323–44.

Spallone, P. (1992) *Generation Games: Genetic Engineering and the Future for Our Lives*, London: Women's Press.

Spallone, P. and Steinberg, L. (eds) (1987) *Made to Order: The Myth of Reproductive and Genetic Progress*, Oxford: Pergamon Press.

Staples, S. (2001) 'Biopicks and biohazards', *Canadian Buisiness*, 19 February: 47–50.

Steinberg, D. L. (1997) *Bodies in Glass: Genetics, Eugenics, Embryo Ethics*, Manchester and New York: Manchester University Press.

Steinberg, D. L. (2000) 'Recombinant bodies: narrative, metaphor and the gene', in S. Williams, J. Gabe and M. Calnan (eds), *Health, Medicine and Society: Key Theories, Future Agendas*, London and New York: Routledge.

Steinbrook, R. (2000) 'Medical journals and medical reporting', *The New England Journal of Medicine*, 342, 22: 1668–71.

Stewart, J., Kendall, E. and Coote, A. (eds) (1994) *Citizens' Juries*, London: Institute for Public Policy Research.

Stock, G. and Campbell, J. (eds) (2000) *Engineering the Human Germline: An Exploration of the Science and Ethics of Altering the Genes We Pass to Our Children*, New York and Oxford: Oxford University Press.

Strathern, M. (1995) 'Nostalgia and the new genetics', in D. Battaglia (ed.) *Rhetorics of Self-Making*, Berkeley, CA: University of California Press.

Strohman, R. (2000) 'Genetic determinism as a failing paradigm in biology and medicine: implications for health and wellness', in M. Schneider Jamner and D. Stokols (eds) *Promoting Human Wellness: New Frontiers for Research, Practice and Policy*, Berkeley, CA: University of California Press.

Sutton, P. (1999) 'Genetics and the future of nature politics', *Sociology Research Online*, 4, 3.

Tagliaferro, L. and Bloom, M. V. (1999) *The Complete Idiot's Guide to Decoding Your Genes*, New York: Alpha.

Tanner, D. (1999) 'Biotechnology enters golden era' (Science and Technology), *The Weekend Australian*, 9–10 October: 12.

Tauli-Corpus, V. (1993) 'We are part of biodiversity, respect our rights', *Third World Resurgence*, 36: 25–6.

Taylor, I. E. (2000) 'Political risk culture: not just a communication failure', in B. Adam, U. Beck and J. Van Loon (eds) *Risk Society and Beyond: Critical Issues for Social Theory*, London: Sage.

Tesh, S. (1988) *Hidden Arguments: Political Ideology and Disease Prevention Policy*, New Brunswick and London: Rutgers University Press.

The Guardian (2000) 'Vaccine in Gm fruit could wipe out hepititis B', *The Guardian*, 8 September.

The Guardian (2000) 'Special report: patenting life', *The Guardian*, 15 November: 1–12.

Theif, K. (2000) 'Celera and NIH's doomed romance', www.doubletwist.com/news/

Thom, D. and Jennings, M. (1999) 'Human pedigree and the "best stock": from eugenics to genetics?', in T. Marteau and M. Richards (eds) *The Troubled Helix: Social and Psychological Implications of the New Human Genetics*, Cambridge: Cambridge University Press.

Titmus, R. M. (1970) *The Gift Relationship*, London: Allen & Unwin.

Turner, B. S. (1992) *Regulating Bodies*, London and New York: Routledge.

Turner, B. S. (1995) *Medical Knowledge and Social Power*, 2nd edition, London: Sage.

Turney, J. (1998) *Frankenstein's Footsteps: Science, Genetics and Popular Culture*, New Haven: Yale University Press.

United Nations (1998) United Nations Development Programme. Overview of *Human Development Report 1997*, www.undp.org/undp/hdro/e98ober/htm

Uzogara, S. G. (2000) 'The impact of genetic modification of human foods in the 21st century', *Biotechnology Advances*, 18 (3 May).

Van Dijck, J. (1998) *Imagenation: Popular Images of Genetics*, New York: New York University Press.

Venter, C. and Cohen, D. (1997) 'Genetic code-breakers', *The Weekend Australian*, 19–20 July: 28.

Waldby, C. (1996) *Aids and the Body Politic*, London and New York: Routledge.

Walford, D. (1994) *The Developed World: Health Policy and Technological Innovation*, J. Newson-Davis and D.J. Weatherall (eds) London: Chapman and Hall.

Walker, A. P. (1998) 'The practice of genetic counselling', in D. L. Baker, J. L. Schuette and W. R. Uhlmann (eds) *A Guide to Genetic Counseling*, New York: Wiley-Liss.

Warwick, H. (2000) 'Terminator too', *The Ecologist* 30, 3: 50

Webler, T. and Renn, O. (1995) 'A brief primer on participation: philosophy and practice', in O. Renn, T. Webler and P. Wiedmann (eds) *Fairness and Competence in Citizen Participation: Evaluating Models of Environmental Discourse*, Dordrecht: Kluwer Academic Publishers.

Webster, G. and Goodwin, B. (1997) *Form and Transformation*, Cambridge: Cambridge University Press.

Wertz, D. C. (1999) 'Patients' and professionals' views on autonomy, disability, and "discrimination": results of a 36-nation survey', in T. A. Caulfield and B. Williams-Jones (eds) *The Commercialization of Genetic Research: Ethical, Legal, and Policy Issues*, Dordrecht: Kluwer Academic/Plenum Publishers.

Wheale, P., von Schomberg, R. and Glasner, P. (eds) (1998) *The Social Management of Genetic Engineering*, Aldershot: Ashgate.

Whimster, S. and Lash, S. (eds) (1987) *Max Weber, Rationality and Modernity*, London: Allen & Unwin.

White, M. T. (1999) 'Making responsible decisions: an interpretive ethic for genetic decisionmaking', *Hastings Center Report*, 29, 1: 14–21.

Whitman, D. B. (2000) 'Genetically modified foods: harmful or helpful?' *Cambridge Scientific Abstracts*, www.csa.com/hottopics/gmfood/overview.html

Whitt, L. A. (1998) 'Biocolonialism and the commodification of knowledge', *Science as Culture*, 7, 1: 33–67.

WHO (1986) *Ottawa Charter for Health Promotion*, Canada: WHO.

WHO (1988) *The Adelaide Recommendations: Healthy Public Policy*, Copenhagen: WHO/EURO.

WHO (1991) 'To create supportive environments for health', *The Sundsvall Handbook*, Geneva: The World Health Organization.

WHO (1997) *Health and Environment in Sustainable Devlopment, 5 Years on After the Earth Summit*, Geneva: The World Health Organization.

Wijeratna, A. (2000) *ActionAid Citizens' Jury Initiative: Indian Farmers Judge GM Crops*, London: ActionAid.

Wilkinson, R. G. (1996) *Unhealthy Societies: The Afflictions of Inequality*, London and New York: Routledge.

Williams, R. (1976) *Keywords: A Vocabulary of Culture and Society*, Glasgow: Fontana/Croom Helm.

Willis, E. (1998) 'Public health, private genes: the social context of genetic biotechnologies', *Critical Public Health*, 8, 2: 131–9.

Wilmut, I., Campbell, K. and Tudge, C. (2000) *The Second Creation: The Age of Biological Control by the Scientists Who Cloned Dolly*, London: Headline.

Wingerson, L. (1998) *Unnatural Selection: The Promise and the Power of Human Genetic Research*, New York: Bantam Books.

Winslow, C. E. (1920) 'The untilled fields of public health', *Science*, 51: 23–33.

Woodford, J. (1999) 'Scientists urge cloning for spare human body parts', *The Sydney Morning Herald*, 17 March: 1.

World Commission on Environment and Development (1987) *Our Common Future (The Brundtland Report)*, New York: WCED.

Zielinski-Gutierrez, E. C. and Kendall, C. (2000) 'The globalization of health and disease: the health transition and global change', in G. Albrecht, R. Fitzpatrick and S. C. Scrimshaw (eds) *Handbook of Social Studies in Health and Medicine*, London: Sage.

Zierler, S. and Krieger, N. (1998) 'HIV infection in women: social inequalities as determinants of risk', *Critical Public Health*, 8, 1: 13–32.

Zilinskas, R. A. and Balint, P. J. (2001) *The Human Genome Project and Minority Communities: Ethical, Social, and Political Dilemmas*, New York: Praeger Publishers.

Zimmern, R. (1999) 'Genetics', in S. Griffiths and D. J. Hunter (eds) *Perspectives in Public Health*, Oxon: Radcliffe Medical Press.

Index

health workers, *au fait* with genetics
52
health-promoting regimens, 'techniques of the self' 83
hepatitis B, vaccine in GM fruit 96
Hepburn, L. 139, 144–5, 203
herbicides 172
Hereditary Disease Unit (Australia)
63
HGDP 32, 164–5, 169, 179
HGP 2, 8, 15–16, 31, 50, 59; counselling as result of 136;
discoveries arising from 113;
'Holy Grail' 117; implications of
118; information from 192; the
media and 103; race for
complete gene map 159; tests
and 63; Western scientists 170
Hickman, B. 18, 113, 116
Hilgartner, S. 108–9
Hill, S. 69, 199, 204
Hippocrates 74, 88
HIV 131
HIV/AIDS 161
Ho, M.W. 93, 97–8
Holtzman, N.A. 20, 153–4
homophobia 195
homosexuals 5, 11, 63, 83, 206
Horgan, J. 5, 46
hospital curative medicine 99
'hot-line' support care 168
House of Lords Select Committee
investigation, DNA data banks
27
House of Lords Select Committee
on Science and Technology
report 185
Hoy, A. 127–8
Hubbard, R. 111, 116
human cloning, responses to 128,
130
human endeavour, climatic change
and nuclear fall-out 90; 'ecocentric approach to environment 93

Human Genetics Commission
(HGC) inquiry, DNA data
banks 27–8
Human Genetics Programme
(HGP) 53
Human Genome Diversity Project
see HGDP
Human Genome Epidemiology
Network (HuGE Net) 53
Human Genome Project *see* HGP
human manipulation, environment
and host 91
Huntington Disease Society of
America 193
Huntington's disease 62, 156
Hygeia 75
hygienic measures, physical environ-
ment and 11
hysterical woman 206

Iceland 117; data base of whole
population 27, 166–7
Iceland Biobanks Act (2000) 166
identity politics, limitations of 206
immigration policy, degenerationist
and hereditarian theories 101;
eugenics and 101
Immunity 115
India 54, 177; Bhopal incident 175;
Citizens' jury and GM crops 190
Indian Department of
Biotechnology 190
individual, responsible for
managing disease 65
individualized market choice, germline engineering and 8
inequalities, counsellor and counsellee 141; uptake of genetic
knowledge and 4, 32, 66
infectious diseases 44, 88, 96–7
information, difficulties in interpreting 58–9; distinction
between genetic and non-
genetic 137; empowering 6, 24;